CONTENTS

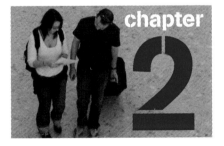

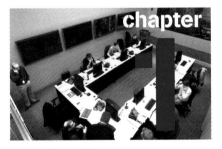

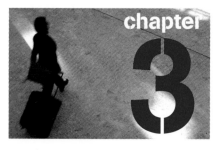

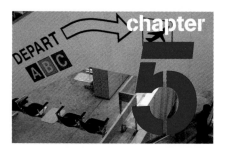

THE WORLD HEALTH REPORT 2007

A SAFER FUTURE

GLOBAL PUBLIC HEALTH SECURITY IN THE 21ST CENTURY

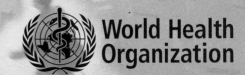

World Health
Organization

WHO Library Cataloguing-in-Publication Data

World Health Organization.
The world health report 2007 : a safer future : global public health security in the 21st century.

1.World health – trends. 2.Disease outbreaks – prevention and control. 3.Legislation, Health. 4.International cooperation.
5.Environmental health. I.Title. II.Title: A safer future: global public health security in the 21st century.

ISBN 978 92 4 156344 4   (NLM classification: WA 530.1)
ISSN 1020-3311

Information concerning this publication can be obtained from:
World Health Report
World Health Organization
1211 Geneva 27, Switzerland
E-mail: whr@who.int

614.42

Copies of this publication can be ordered from: bookorders@who.int

This report was produced under the leadership of Director-General, Margaret Chan. David Heymann, Assistant Director-General for
Communicable Diseases, was Editor-in-Chief. The main writers were Thomson Prentice and Lina Tucker Reinders of the World Health Report
team.

Advice and support were gratefully received from all Assistant Directors-General, Regional Directors, numerous WHO technical units, and many
others who reviewed and contributed to the text.

Special thanks for their contributions are due to Tomas Allen, Penelope Andrea, Bruce Aylward, Anand Balachandran, Sona Bari, Diarmid
Campbell-Lendrum, Amina Chaieb, Claire Lise Chaignat, May Chu, Albert Concha-Eastman, Ottorino Cosivi, Alvaro Cruz, Kevin De Cock,Sophia
Desillas, Pat Drury, Pierre Formenty, Keiji Fukuda, Fernando Gonzalez–Martin, Pascal Haefliger, Max Hardiman, Mary Kay Kindhauser, Colin
Mathers, Angela Merianos, Francois-Xavier Meslin, Michael Nathan, Maria Neira, Paul Nunn, Kevin O'Reilly, Andrée Pinard-Clark, Guenael
Rodier, Oliver Rosenbauer, Cathy Roth, Mike Ryan, Jorgen Schlundt, George Schmid, Ian Smith, Claudia Stein and Leo Vita-Finzi.

The report was edited by Diana Hopkins, assisted by Barbara Campanini. Figures, tables and other illustrations were provided by Gael Kernen,
who also produced the web site version and other electronic media. Vreni Schoenenberger assisted in historical research. Administrative
support to the World Health Report team was provided by Saba Amdeselassie. The index was prepared by June Morrison.

Photo credits: Agence France-Presse/Paula Bronstein (pp. viii, 34); International Federation of the Red Cross and Red Crescent Societies (IFRC)/
Christopher Black (p. 25); IFRC/Marko Kokic (p. 22); United Nations Integrated Regional Information Networks (IRIN) (p. 41); Jean-Pierre Revel
(p. 30); United States National Library of Medicine (NLM) (p. 47); WHO/Olivier Asselin (pp. viii, 16); WHO/Christopher Black (pp. viii, xiv, xvi,
xviii, xx, xxii, 1, 16, 34, 44, 56, 64); WHO/Christopher Black, Chris de Bode, Umit Kartoglu, Marko Kokic and Jean Mohr (cover); WHO/Chris de
Bode (p. 19); WHO/Marko Kokic (pp. 20, 21); WHO/Jean Mohr (pp. viii, 1).

Illustrations: The Plague Doctor, unknown artist, Wellcome Library, London (p. 2); Death's Dispensary, George Pinwell, 1866 (p. 4); Edward
Jenner Performing the First Vaccination against Smallpox in 1796, Gaston Melingue, 1879, Bibliothèque de l'Académie nationale de Médecine,
Paris (p. 5).

Design: Reda Sadki
Layout: Steve Ewart and Reda Sadki
Figures: Christophe Grangier
Printing Coordination: Raphaël Crettaz
Printed in France

Figures – Chapters

Boxes – Chapters

Tables – Chapters

vi

world health report 2007
global public health security
in the 21st century

The world has changed dramatically since 1951, when WHO issued its first set of legally binding regulations aimed at preventing the international spread of disease. At that time, the disease situation was relatively stable. Concern focused on only six "quarantinable" diseases: cholera, plague, relapsing fever, smallpox, typhus and yellow fever. New diseases were rare, and miracle drugs had revolutionized the care of many well-known infections. People travelled internationally by ship, and news travelled by telegram.

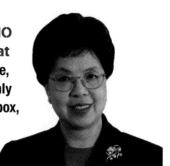

MESSAGE
FROM THE DIRECTOR-GENERAL

Since then, profound changes have occurred in the way humanity inhabits the planet. The disease situation is anything but stable. Population growth, incursion into previously uninhabited areas, rapid urbanization, intensive farming practices, environmental degradation, and the misuse of antimicrobials have disrupted the equilibrium of the microbial world. New diseases are emerging at the historically unprecedented rate of one per year. Airlines now carry more than 2 billion passengers annually, vastly increasing opportunities for the rapid international spread of infectious agents and their vectors.

Dependence on chemicals has increased, as has awareness of the potential hazards for health and the environment. Industrialization of food production and processing, and globalization of marketing and distribution mean that a single tainted ingredient can lead to the recall of tons of food items from scores of countries. In a particularly ominous trend, mainstay antimicrobials are failing at a rate that outpaces the development of replacement drugs.

These threats have become a much larger menace in a world characterized by high mobility, economic interdependence and electronic interconnectedness. Traditional defences at national borders cannot protect against the invasion of a disease or vector. Real time news allows panic to spread with equal ease. Shocks to health reverberate as shocks to economies and business continuity in areas well beyond the affected site. Vulnerability is universal.

The *World Health Report 2007* is dedicated to promoting global public health security – the reduced vulnerability of populations to acute threats to health. This year's World Health Day, celebrated in April, launched WHO's discussion on global public health security. Around the world, academics, students, health professionals, politicians and the business community are engaged in dialogue on how to protect the world from threats like pandemic influenza, the health consequences of conflict and natural disasters, and bioterrorism.

The *World Health Report 2007* addresses these issues, among others, in the context of new tools for collective defence, including, most notably, the revised International Health Regulations (2005). These Regulations are an international legal instrument designed to achieve maximum security against the international spread of diseases. They also aim to reduce the international impact of public health emergencies.

The IHR (2005) expand the focus of collective defence from just a few "quarantinable" diseases to include any emergency with international repercussions for health, including outbreaks of emerging and epidemic-prone diseases, outbreaks of foodborne disease, natural disasters, and chemical or radionuclear events, whether accidental or caused deliberately.

In a significant departure from the past, IHR (2005) move away from a focus on passive barriers at borders, airports and seaports to a strategy of proactive risk management. This strategy aims to detect an event early and stop it at its source – before it has a chance to become an international threat.

Given today's universal vulnerability to these threats, better security calls for global solidarity. International public health security is both a collective aspiration and a mutual responsibility. As the determinants and consequences of health emergencies have become broader, so has the range of players with a stake in the security agenda. The new watchwords are diplomacy, cooperation, transparency and preparedness. Successful implementation of IHR (2005) serves the interests of politicians and business leaders as well as the health, trade and tourism sectors.

I am pleased to present the *World Health Report 2007* to our partners and look forward to the discussions, directions and actions that it will inspire.

Dr Margaret Chan
Director-General
World Health Organization

viii

world health report 2007
global public health security
in the 21st century

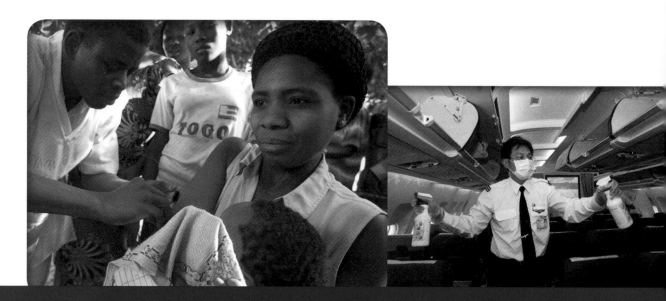

OVERVIEW

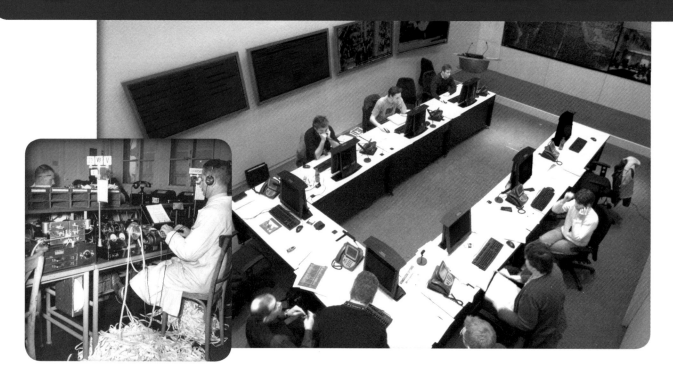

At a time when the world faces many new and recurring threats, the ambitious aim of this year's *World Health Report* is to show how collective international public health action can build a safer future for humanity.

This is the overall goal of global public health security. For the purposes of this report, global public health security is defined as the activities required, both proactive and reactive, to minimize vulnerability to acute public health events that endanger the collective health of populations living across geographical regions and international boundaries.

As the events illustrated in this report show, global health security, or the lack of it, may also have an impact on economic or political stability, trade, tourism, access to goods and services

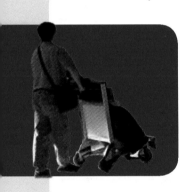

and, if they occur repeatedly, on demographic stability. It embraces a wide range of complex and daunting issues, from the international stage to the individual household, including the health consequences of poverty, wars and conflicts, climate change, natural catastrophes and man-made disasters.

All of these are areas of continuing WHO work and will be the topics of forthcoming publications. The 2008 World Health Report, for example, will be concerned with individual health security, concentrating on the role of primary health care and humanitarian action in providing access to the essential prerequisites for health.

This report, however, focuses on specific issues that threaten the collective health of people internationally: infectious disease epidemics, pandemics and other acute health events as defined by the revised International Health Regulations, known as IHR (2005), which came into force in June of this year.

The purpose of these Regulations is to prevent the spread of disease across international borders. They are a vital legislative instrument of global public health security, providing the necessary global framework to prevent, detect, assess and, if necessary, provide a coordinated response to events that may constitute a public health emergency of international concern.

Meeting the requirements in the revised IHR (2005) is a challenge that requires time, commitment and the willingness to change. The Regulations are broader and more demanding than those they replace, with a much greater emphasis on the responsibility of all countries to have in place effective systems for detection and control of public health risks – and to accomplish this by 2012.

A strategic plan has been developed by WHO to guide countries in the implementation of the obligations in the Regulations and to help them overcome the inherent challenges.

GLOBAL PUBLIC HEALTH THREATS IN THE 21ST CENTURY

Today's highly mobile, interdependent and interconnected world provides myriad opportunities for the rapid spread of infectious diseases, and radionuclear and toxic threats, which is why updated and expanded Regulations are necessary. Infectious diseases are now spreading geographically much faster than at any time in history. It is estimated that 2.1 billion airline passengers travelled in 2006; an outbreak or epidemic in any one part of the world is only a few hours away from becoming an imminent threat somewhere else (see Figure 1).

Infectious diseases are not only spreading faster, they appear to be emerging more quickly than ever before. Since the 1970s, newly emerging diseases have been identified at the unprecedented rate of one or more per year. There are now nearly 40 diseases that were unknown a generation ago. In addition, during the last five years, WHO has verified more than 1100 epidemic events worldwide.

The categories and examples given below illustrate the variety and breadth of public health threats confronting people today.

Epidemic-prone diseases

Cholera, yellow fever and epidemic meningococcal diseases made a comeback in the last quarter of the 20th century and call for renewed efforts in surveillance, prevention and control. Severe Acute Respiratory Syndrome (SARS) and avian influenza in humans have triggered major international concern, raised new scientific challenges, caused major human suffering and imposed enormous economic damage. Other emerging viral diseases such as Ebola, Marburg haemorrhagic fever and Nipah virus pose threats to global public health security and also require containment at their source due to their acute nature and resulting illness and mortality. During outbreaks of these diseases, rapid assessment and response, often needing international assistance, has been required to limit local spread. Strengthening of capacity is imperative in the future to assess such new threats.

Figure 1   Verified events of potential international public health concern, by WHO region, September 2003–September 2006

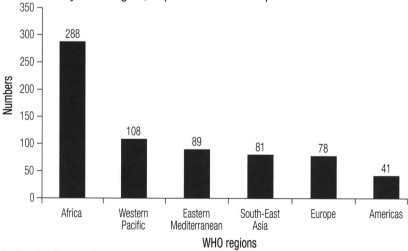

Total number of cases = 685

Gains in many areas of infectious disease control are seriously jeopardized by the spread of antimicrobial resistance, with extensively drug-resistant tuberculosis (XDR-TB) now a cause of great concern. Drug resistance is also evident in diarrhoeal diseases, hospital-acquired infections, malaria, meningitis, respiratory tract infections, and sexually transmitted infections, and is emerging in HIV.

Foodborne diseases

The food chain has undergone considerable and rapid changes over the last 50 years, becoming highly sophisticated and international. Although the safety of food has dramatically improved overall, progress is uneven and foodborne outbreaks from microbial contamination, chemicals and toxins are common in many countries. The trading of contaminated food between countries increases the potential that outbreaks will spread. In addition, the emergence of new foodborne diseases creates considerable concern, such as the recognition of the new variant of Creutzfeldt-Jakob disease (vCJD) associated with bovine spongiform encephalopathy (BSE).

Accidental and deliberate outbreaks

As activities related to infectious disease surveillance and laboratory research have increased in recent years, so too has the potential for outbreaks associated with the accidental release of infectious agents. Breaches in biosafety measures are often responsible for these accidents. At the same time, opportunities for malicious releases of dangerous pathogens, once unthinkable, have become a reality, as shown by the anthrax letters in the United States of America in 2001.

In addition, the recent past has been marked by disturbing new health events that resulted from chemical or nuclear accidents and sudden environmental changes, causing major concerns in many parts of the world.

Toxic chemical accidents

■ West Africa, 2006: the dumping of approximately 500 tons of petrochemical waste in at least 15 sites around the city of Abidjan, Côte d'Ivoire, led to the deaths of eight people being attributed to exposure to the waste and to nearly 90 000 more people seeking medical help. Other countries were concerned that they could also have been put at risk as a result of dumping elsewhere or as a result of chemical contamination of transboundary rivers.

■ Southern Europe, 1981: 203 people died after consuming poisoned cooking oil that was adulterated with industrial rapeseed oil. A total of 15 000 people were affected by the tainted oil and no cure to reverse the adverse effects of toxic oil syndrome was ever found.

Radionuclear accidents

■ Eastern Europe, 1986: the Chernobyl disaster is regarded as the worst accident in the history of nuclear power. The explosion at the plant resulted in the radioactive contamination of the surrounding geographical area, and a cloud of radioactive fallout drifted over western parts of the former Soviet Union, eastern and western Europe, some Nordic countries and eastern North America. Large areas of Ukraine, the Republic of Belarus and the Russian Federation were badly contaminated, resulting in the evacuation and resettlement of over 336 000 people.

xii

world health report 2007
global public health security
in the 21st century

Environmental disasters

- Europe, 2003: the heatwave in Europe that claimed the lives of 35 000 persons was linked to unprecedented extremes in weather in other parts of the world during the same period.
- Central Africa, 1986: more than 1700 people died of carbon dioxide poisoning following a massive release of gas from Lake Nyos, a volcanic crater lake. Such an event requires rapid assessment to determine if it is an international threat.

This Overview summarizes some of the above examples, which, together with the lessons drawn from them, are more widely discussed in the report. The report emphasizes that the international response required today is not only to the known, but also to the unknown – the diseases that may arise from acute environmental or climatic changes and from industrial pollution and accidents that may put millions of people at risk in several countries.

GLOBAL COLLABORATION TO MEET THREATS TO PUBLIC HEALTH SECURITY

These threats require urgent action, and WHO and its partners have much to offer immediately as well as in the longer term. This is an area where real progress to protect whole populations can be made, starting now. It is also where recent history shows that some of the most serious threats to human existence are likely to emerge without warning. It would be extremely naïve and complacent to assume that there will not be another disease like AIDS, another Ebola, or another SARS, sooner or later.

A more secure world that is ready and prepared to respond collectively in the face of threats to global health security requires global partnerships that bring together all countries and stakeholders in all relevant sectors, gather the best technical support and mobilize the necessary resources for effective and timely implementation of IHR (2005). This calls for national core capacity in disease detection and international collaboration for public health emergencies of international concern.

While many of these partnerships are already in place, there are serious gaps, particularly in the health systems of many countries, which weaken the consistency

Figure 2   Global outbreaks, the challenge: late reporting and response

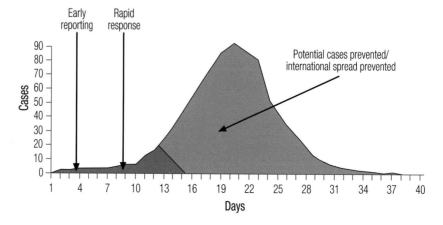

of global health collaboration. In order to compensate for these gaps, an effective global system of epidemic alert and response was initiated by WHO in 1996. It was built essentially on a concept of international partnership with many other agencies and technical institutions. Systematic mechanisms for gathering epidemic intelligence and verifying the existence of outbreaks were established and prompted risk assessments, information dissemination and rapid field response. Regional and global mechanisms for stockpiling and rapid distribution of vaccines, drugs and specialized investigation and protection equipment were also established for public health events caused by haemorrhagic fevers, influenza, meningitis, smallpox and yellow fever.

Today, the public health security of all countries depends on the capacity of each to act effectively and contribute to the security of all. The world is rapidly changing and nothing today moves faster than information. This makes the sharing of essential health information one of the most feasible routes to global public health security.

Instant electronic communication means that disease outbreaks can no longer be kept secret, as was often the case during the implementation of the previous International Health Regulations (1969), known as IHR (1969). Governments were unwilling to report outbreaks because of the potential damage to their economies through disruptions in trade, travel and tourism. In reality, rumours are more damaging than facts. Trust is built through transparency, and trust is necessary for international cooperation in health and development (see Figure 2).

The first steps that must be taken towards global public health security, therefore, are to develop core detection and response capacities in all countries, and to maintain new levels of cooperation between countries to reduce the risks to public health security outlined above. This entails countries strengthening their health systems and ensuring they have the capacity to prevent and control epidemics that can quickly spread across borders and even across continents. Where countries are unable to achieve prevention and control by themselves, it means providing rapid, expert international disease surveillance and response networks to assist them – and making sure these mesh together into an efficient safety net. Above all, it means all countries conforming to and benefiting from IHR (2005).

world health report 2007
xiv global public health security
in the 21st century

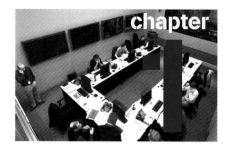

CHAPTER SUMMARIES

Evolution of public health security

Chapter 1 begins by tracing some of the first steps, historically, that led to the introduction of IHR (1969) – landmarks in public health starting with quarantine, a term coined in the 14th century and employed as a protection against "foreign" diseases such as plague; improvements in sanitation that were effective in controlling cholera outbreaks in the 19th century; and the advent of vaccination which led to the eradication of smallpox and the control of many other infectious diseases in the 20th century. Understanding the history of international health cooperation – its successes and its failures – is essential in appreciating its new relevance and potential.

Numerous international conferences on disease control in the late 19th and early 20th centuries led to the foundation of WHO in 1948. In 1951, WHO Member States adopted the International Sanitary Regulations, which were replaced and renamed the International Health Regulations in 1969. Starting in 1995, the Regulations were revised through an intergovernmental process which took into account new epidemiological understanding and accumulated experience, and which responded to the changing world and the related increased threats to global public health security. It was agreed that a code of conduct was required that could not only prevent and control such threats, but could also provide a public health response to them while avoiding unnecessary interference with international trade and traffic. The revision process was completed in 2005 and the Regulations are now referred to as IHR (2005).

Chapter 1 describes how the basis of an effective global system of epidemic alert and response was initiated by WHO in 1996 and how it has been widely expanded since then. It was built essentially on a concept of international partnership with many other agencies and technical institutions. Called the Global Outbreak Alert and Response Network (GOARN), this partnership provides an operational and coordination framework to access expertise and skill, and to keep the international community constantly alert to the threat of outbreaks and ready to respond. Coordinated by WHO, the network is made up of over 140 technical partners from more than 60 countries.

In addition, the unique, large-scale active surveillance network developed by the Global Polio Eradication Initiative is being used to support surveillance of many other vaccine-preventable diseases, such as measles, meningitis, neonatal tetanus and yellow fever. This network is also regularly supporting outbreak surveillance and response activities for other health emergencies and outbreaks described in the report. In 2002, WHO established the Chemical Incident Alert and Response System to operate along similar lines to GOARN. This was extended in 2006 to cover other environmental health emergencies, including those related to the disruption of environmental health services, such as water supply and sanitation, as well as radiological events and emergencies.

The revised Regulations define an emergency as an "extraordinary event" that could spread internationally or might require a coordinated international response. Events that may constitute a public health emergency of international concern are assessed by State Parties using a decision instrument and, if particular criteria are met, WHO must be notified. Mandatory notification is called for in a single case of a disease that could threaten global public health security: human influenza caused by a new virus subtype, poliomyelitis caused by a wild-type poliovirus, SARS and smallpox.

The broad definitions of "public health emergency of international concern" and "disease" allow for the inclusion in IHR (2005) of threats beyond infectious diseases, including those caused by the accidental or intentional release of pathogens, or chemical or radionuclear materials. This extends the scope of the Regulations to protect global public health security in a comprehensive way.

The IHR (2005) redirect the focus from an almost exclusive concentration on measures at airports and seaports aimed at blocking the importation of cases, as required in IHR (1969), towards a rapid response at the source of an outbreak. They introduce a set of "core capacity requirements" that all countries must meet in order to detect, assess, notify and report the events covered by IHR (2005) and aim to strengthen collaboration on a global scale by seeking to improve capacity and demonstrate to countries that compliance is in their best interests. Thus, compliance has three compelling incentives: to reduce the disruptive consequences of an outbreak, to speed its containment, and to maintain good standing in the eyes of the international community.

A revolutionary departure from previous international conventions and regulations is the fact that IHR (2005) explicitly acknowledges that non-state sources of information about outbreaks will often pre-empt official notifications. This includes situations where countries may be reluctant to reveal an event in their territories. WHO is now authorized through IHR (2005) to take into account information sources other than official notifications. WHO will always seek official verification of such information from the country involved before taking any action based on the information received. This reflects a new reality in a world of instant communications: the concealment of disease outbreaks is no longer a viable option for governments.

xvi

world health report 2007
global public health security
in the 21st century

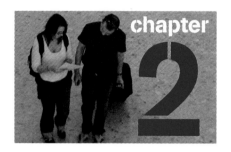

Threats to public health security

Chapter 2 explores a range of threats to global public health security, as defined by IHR (2005), which result from human actions or causes, from human interaction with the environment, and from sudden chemical and radioactive events, including industrial accidents and natural phenomena. It begins by illustrating how inadequate investment in public health, resulting from a false sense of security in the absence of infectious disease outbreaks, has led to reduced vigilance and a relaxing of adherence to effective prevention programmes.

For example, following the widespread use of insecticides in large-scale, systematic control programmes, by the late 1960s most of the important vector-borne diseases were no longer considered major public health problems outside of sub-Saharan Africa. Control programmes then lapsed as resources dwindled. The result was that within the next 20 years, many important vector-borne diseases including African trypanosomiasis, dengue and dengue haemorrhagic fever, and malaria emerged in new areas or re-emerged in areas previously affected. Urbanization and increasing international trade and travel have contributed to rapid spread of dengue viruses and their vectors. Dengue caused an unprecedented pandemic in 1998, with 1.2 million cases reported to WHO from 56 countries. Since then, dengue epidemics have continued, affecting millions of people from Latin America to South-East Asia. Globally, the average annual number of cases reported to WHO has nearly doubled in each of the last four decades.

Inadequate surveillance results from a lack of commitment to build effective health systems capable of monitoring a country's health status. The rapid global emergence and spread of HIV/AIDS in the 1970s illustrates this. The presence of this new health threat was not detected by what were invariably weak health systems in many developing countries. It only belatedly became a matter of international concern with the first cases in the United States. In addition to limited disease surveillance capacity and data, early efforts to control the AIDS epidemic were also hampered by a lack of solid data on sexual behaviour in African countries, the United States and other industrialized countries. Behavioural data were practically non-existent in the developing world. The understanding of HIV/AIDS in the context of sexuality, gender relations and migration in the developing world took years to develop and is still poorly understood.

Even with reliable operations in place, other influences on public health programmes can have lethal and costly repercussions. Such was the case in August 2003, when unsubstantiated claims originating in northern Nigeria that the oral poliomyelitis vaccine (OPV) was unsafe and could sterilize young children led to the suspension of polio immunization in two northern states and substantial reductions in polio immunization coverage in a number of others. The result was a large outbreak of polio across northern Nigeria and the reinfection of previously polio-free areas in the south of the country. This outbreak eventually paralysed thousands of children in Nigeria and spread from northern Nigeria to 19 polio-free countries.

Chapter 2 also considers the public health consequences of conflicts, such as the outbreak of Marburg haemorrhagic fever against the background of the 1975-2002 civil war in Angola, and the cholera epidemic in the Democratic Republic of the Congo in the aftermath of the crisis in Rwanda in 1994. In July of that year, between 500 000 and 800 000 people crossed the border to seek refuge in the outskirts of the Congolese city of Goma. During the first month after their arrival, close to 50 000 refugees died in a widespread outbreak of combined cholera and shigella dysentery. The speed of transmission and the high rate of infection were related to the contamination with *Vibrio cholerae* of the only available source of water and the absence of proper housing and sanitation.

The problem of microbial adaptation, the use and misuse of antibiotics and zoonotic diseases, such as human bovine spongiform encephalopathy (BSE) and Nipah virus, is discussed. The history of Nipah virus emergence provides another example of a new human pathogen that originated from an animal source, initially caused zoonotic disease, and subsequently evolved to become a more efficient human pathogen. This trend calls for closer collaboration among sectors responsible for human health, veterinary health and wildlife.

Infectious diseases following extreme weather-related events and the acute public health impact of sudden chemical and radioactive events are also discussed. These now fall within the scope of IHR (2005) if they have the potential to cause harm on an international scale, including the deliberate use of biological and chemical agents, and industrial accidents. Among the examples of accidents given here is the Chernobyl nuclear accident in Ukraine in 1986, which dispersed radioactive materials into the atmosphere over a huge area of Europe. Put together, the examples in this chapter reveal the alarming variety of threats to global health security towards the end of the 20th century.

xviii

world health report 2007
global public health security
in the 21st century

chapter

3

New health threats in the 21st century

Chapter 3 examines three new health threats that have emerged in the 21st century – bioterrorism in the form of the anthrax letters in the United States in 2001, the emergence of SARS in 2003, and the large-scale dumping of toxic chemical waste in Côte d'Ivoire in 2006.

Coming only days after the terrorist events of 11 September 2001, the deliberate dissemination of potentially lethal anthrax spores in letters sent through the United States Postal Service added bioterrorism to the realities of life in modern society. In addition to the human toll – five died out of a total of 22 people affected – the anthrax attack had huge economic, public health and security consequences. It prompted renewed international concerns about bioterrorism, provoking countermeasures in many countries and requests for a greater advisory role by WHO led to the updating of the publication *Public health response to biological and chemical weapons: WHO guidance*.

The anthrax letters showed the potential of bioterrorism to cause not just death and disability, but enormous social and economic disruption. A simultaneous worry was that smallpox – eradicated as a human disease in 1979 – could be used over 20 years later to deadly effect in deliberate acts of violence. Mass smallpox vaccination had been discontinued after eradication, thus leaving unimmunized populations susceptible and a new generation of public health practitioners without clinical experience of the disease.

Since then, WHO has taken part in international discussions and bioterrorism desktop exercises arguing that the surest way to detect a deliberately caused outbreak is by strengthening the systems used for detecting and responding to natural outbreaks, as the epidemiological and laboratory principles are fundamentally the same. Expert discussions on the appropriate response to a biological attack, especially with the smallpox virus, served to test – on a global scale – the outbreak alert and response mechanisms already introduced by WHO.

In 2003, SARS – the first severe new disease of this century – confirmed fears, generated by the bioterrorism threat, that a new or unfamiliar pathogen might have profound national and international implications for public health and economic security. SARS defined the features that would give a disease international significance as a global public health security threat: it spread from person to person, required no vector, displayed no particular geographical affinity, incubated silently for more than a week, mimicked the symptoms of many other diseases, took its heaviest toll on hospital staff, and killed around 10% of those infected. These features meant that it spread easily along the routes of international air travel, placing every city with an international airport at risk of imported cases.

New, deadly and – initially – poorly understood, SARS incited a degree of public anxiety that virtually halted travel to affected areas and drained billions of dollars from economies across entire regions. It challenged public and political perceptions of the risks associated with emerging and epidemic-prone diseases and raised the profile of public health to new heights. Not every country felt threatened by the prospect of bioterrorism, but every country was concerned by the arrival of a disease like SARS.

It showed that the danger arising from emerging diseases is universal. No country, rich or poor, is adequately protected from either the arrival of a new disease on its territory or the subsequent disruption this can cause. The spread of SARS was halted less than four months after it was first recognized as an international threat – an unprecedented achievement for public health on a global scale. If SARS had become permanently established as yet another indigenous epidemic threat, it is not difficult to imagine the consequences for global public health security in a world still struggling to cope with HIV/AIDS.

As well as the international mobility of people, the global movement of products can have serious health consequences. The potentially deadly risks of the international movement and disposal of hazardous wastes as an element of global trade were vividly illustrated in Côte d'Ivoire in August 2006. Over 500 tons of chemical waste were unloaded from a cargo ship and illegally dumped by trucks at different sites in and around Abidjan. As a result, almost 90 000 people sought medical treatment in the following days and weeks. Although less than 100 people were hospitalized and far fewer deaths could be attributed to the event, it was a public health crisis of both national and international dimensions. One of the main international concerns was that the cargo ship had sailed from northern Europe and had called at a number of ports, including some others in western Africa, on its way to Côte d'Ivoire. It was unclear in the aftermath of the incident whether it had taken on, or discharged, chemical waste at any of those ports of call.

world health report 2007
global public health security
in the 21st century

XX

chapter

4

Learning lessons, thinking ahead

Chapter 4 is devoted to potential public health emergencies of international concern, the most feared of which remains pandemic influenza. The response to this threat has already been proactive – facilitated by early implementation of IHR (2005). This has been a rare opportunity to prepare for a pandemic, and possibly to prevent the threat becoming a reality by taking full advantage of advance warning and by testing a model for pandemic planning and preparedness. This advantage must be fully exploited to enhance global preparedness within the framework of IHR (2005).

Coming on the heels of the SARS outbreak, the prospect of an influenza pandemic sparked immediate alarm around the world. Far more contagious, spread by coughing and sneezing and transmissible within an incubation period too short to allow for contact tracing and isolation, pandemic influenza would have devastating consequences. If a fully transmissible pandemic virus emerged, the spread of the disease could not be prevented.

Based on experiences with past pandemics, illness affecting around 25% of the world's population – more than 1.5 billion people – could be anticipated. Even if the influenza pandemic virus caused relatively mild disease, the economic and social disruption arising from sudden surges of illness in so many people would be enormous.

As the next influenza pandemic is likely to be of avian variety, many interventions have been taken to control the initial outbreaks in poultry, including the destruction of tens of millions of birds. Chapter 4 describes the key actions taken and the remarkable degree of international collaboration that has been achieved to reduce the pandemic risk. Among its many front-line activities, WHO has tracked and verified dozens of daily rumours of human cases. Field investigation kits have been dispatched to countries and training on field investigations and response intensified. The GOARN mechanism was mobilized to support the deployment of WHO response teams to 10 countries with H5N1 infection in humans and/or poultry, while over 30 assessment teams investigated the potential H5N1 situation in other countries.

With the aim of promoting global preparedness, WHO developed a strategic action plan for pandemic influenza that set out five key action areas.

- Reducing human exposure to the H5N1 virus.
- Strengthening the early warning system.
- Intensifying rapid containment operations.
- Building capacity to cope with a pandemic.
- Coordinating global scientific research and development.

By May 2007, when 12 countries had reported 308 human cases including 186 deaths, nearly all countries had established avian and human pandemic preparedness plans. Working together, WHO and some Member States created international stockpiles of oseltamivir, an antiviral drug that potentially could stop transmission in an early focus of human-to-human transmission. The pharmaceutical industry continues to search for a pandemic influenza vaccine. In 2007, outbreaks in poultry continued, as did sporadic cases in humans, but a pandemic virus failed to emerge. Nevertheless, scientists agree that the threat of a pandemic from H5N1 continues and that the question of a pandemic of influenza from this virus or another avian influenza virus is still a matter of when, not if.

Chapter 4 also highlights the problem of XDR-TB in southern Africa, exacerbated by inadequate health systems and the resulting failures in programme management, especially poor supervision of health staff and patients' treatment regimens, disruptions in drug supplies, and poor clinical management, all of which can prevent patients completing courses of treatment. The current situation is a wake-up call to all countries, and especially those in Africa, to ensure that basic tuberculosis control reaches international standards and to initiate and strengthen management of drug-resistant forms of the disease.

The 2003-2005 global spread of poliovirus caused by inadequate control in Nigeria (described in Chapter 2) was another wake-up call. It underscored the risk that polio might re-emerge post-eradication and the importance of the designation of polio as a notifiable disease in IHR (2005). The alert and reporting mechanisms mandated by IHR (2005) are an essential complement to activities undertaken by the extensive surveillance network already in place around the world that provides for the immediate notification of confirmed polio cases and for standardized clinical and virologic investigation of potential cases. This capacity to remain alert and to respond is fundamental to the ability to eradicate polio because, once the virus is eradicated in nature, the world will need be vigilant in case of accidental or deliberate release of the virus.

Finally, Chapter 4 considers natural disasters which, in 2006 alone, affected 134.6 million people and killed 21 342 others. Just as these situations endanger individuals, they can also threaten already stressed health systems that people rely on to maintain their personal health security. The indirect effects of natural disasters include the threat of infectious disease epidemics, acute malnutrition, population displacement, acute mental illness and the exacerbation of chronic disease, all of which require strong health systems to deal with them.

xxii

world health report 2007
global public health security
in the 21st century

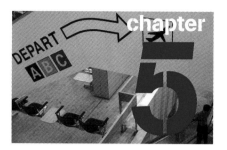

Towards a safer future

Chapter 5 emphasizes the importance of strengthening health systems in building global public health security. It argues that many of the public health emergencies described in this report could have been prevented or better controlled if the health systems concerned had been stronger and better prepared. Some countries find it more difficult than others to confront threats to public health security effectively because they lack the necessary resources, because their health infrastructure has collapsed as a consequence of under-investment and shortages of trained health workers, or because the infrastructure has been damaged or destroyed by armed conflict or a previous natural disaster.

No single country – however capable, wealthy or technologically advanced – can alone prevent, detect and respond to all public health threats. Emerging threats may be unseen from a national perspective, may require a global analysis for proper risk assessment, or may necessitate effective coordination at the international level.

This is the basis for IHR (2005), but as not all countries will be able to take up the challenge immediately, WHO will have to draw upon its long experience as the leader in global public health, its convening power, and its partnerships with governments, United Nations agencies, civil society, academia, the private sector and the media to maintain its surveillance and global alert and response systems.

As described in Chapter 1, WHO surveillance networks and GOARN are effective international partnerships that provide both a service and a safety net. GOARN is able to deploy response teams to any part of the world within 24 hours to provide direct support to national authorities. WHO's various surveillance and laboratory networks are able to capture the global picture of public health risks and assist in efficient case analysis.

Together, these systems fill acute gaps caused by the lack of national capacity and protect the world when there may be a desire to delay reporting for political or other reasons.

The effective maintenance of these systems, however, must be adequately resourced with staff, technology and financial support. The building of national capacity will not diminish the need for WHO's global networks. Rather, increased partnerships, knowledge transfer, advancing technologies, event management and strategic communications will grow as IHR (2005) reaches full implementation.

Conclusions and recommendations

The report concludes with recommendations intended to provide guidance and inspiration towards cooperation and transparency in the effort to secure the highest level of global public health security.

- Full implementation of IHR (2005) by all countries. The protection of national and global public health must be transparent in government affairs, be seen as a cross-cutting issue and as a crucial element integrated into economic and social policies and systems.
- Global cooperation in surveillance and outbreak alert and response between governments, United Nations agencies, private sector industries and organizations, professional associations, academia, media agencies and civil society, building particularly on the eradication of polio to create an effective and comprehensive surveillance and response infrastructure.
- Open sharing of knowledge, technologies and materials, including viruses and other laboratory samples, necessary to optimize secure global public health. The struggle for global public health security will be lost if vaccines, treatment regimens, and facilities and diagnostics are available only to the wealthy.
- Global responsibility for capacity building within the public health infrastructure of all countries. National systems must be strengthened to anticipate and predict hazards effectively both at the international and national levels and to allow for effective preparedness strategies.
- Cross-sector collaboration within governments. The protection of global public health security is dependent on trust and collaboration between sectors such as health, agriculture, trade and tourism. It is for this reason that the capacity to understand and act in the best interests of the intricate relationship between public health security and these sectors must be fostered.
- Increased global and national resources for the training of public health personnel, the advancement of surveillance, the building and enhancing of laboratory capacity, the support of response networks, and the continuation and progression of prevention campaigns.

Although the subject of this report has taken a global approach to public health security, WHO does not neglect the fact that all individuals – women, men and children – are affected by the common threats to health. It is vital not to lose sight of the personal consequences of global health challenges. This was the inspiration that led to the "health for all" commitment to primary health care in 1978. That commitment and the principles supporting it remain untarnished and as essential as ever. On that basis, primary health care and humanitarian action in times of crisis – two means to ensure health security at individual and community levels – will be discussed at length in *The World Health Report 2008*.

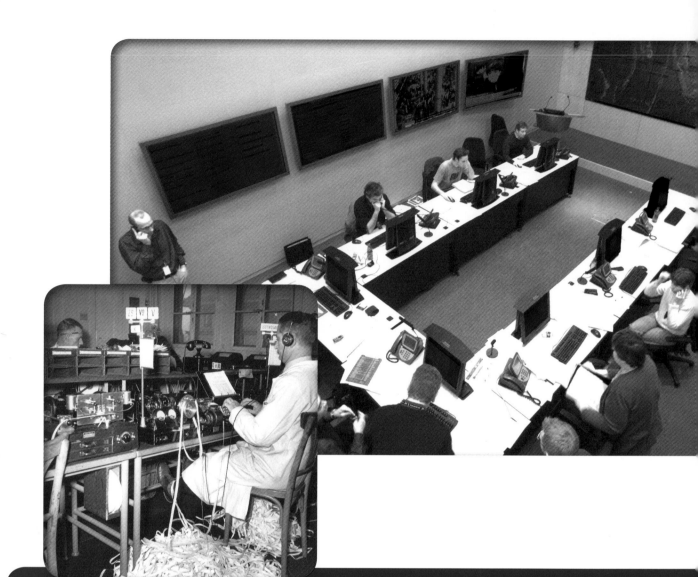

EVOLUTION OF PUBLIC HEALTH
security

Chapter 1 begins by tracing some of the first steps, historically, that led to the introduction of the International Health Regulations (1969) – landmarks in public health starting with quarantine, a term coined in the 14th century and employed as a protection against "foreign" diseases such as plague; improvements in sanitation that were effective in controlling cholera outbreaks in the 19th century; and the advent of vaccination, which led to the eradication of smallpox and the control of many other infectious diseases in the 20th century. Understanding the history of international health cooperation – its successes and its failures – is essential in appreciating its new relevance and potential.

Throughout history, humanity has been challenged by outbreaks of infectious diseases and other health emergencies that have spread, caused death on unprecedented levels and threatened public health security (see Box 1.1). With no better solution, people's response was to remove the sick from the healthy population and wait until the epidemic ran its course.

With time, scientific knowledge evolved, containment measures became more sophisticated and some infectious disease outbreaks were gradually brought under control with improved sanitation and the discovery of vaccines. However, microbial organisms are well-equipped to invade new territories, adapt to new ecological niches or hosts, change their virulence or modes of transmission, and develop resistance to drugs. An organism that can replicate itself a million times within a day clearly has an evolutionary advantage, with chance and surprise on its side. Therefore, no matter how experienced or refined containment measures became over the years, there was always the possibility of another outbreak causing an epidemic anytime, anywhere. The reality is that the battle to keep up with microbial evolution and adaptation will never be won.

Box 1.1 Public health security

Public health security is defined as the activities required, both proactive and reactive, to minimize vulnerability to acute public health events that endanger the collective health of national populations.

Global public health security widens this definition to include acute public health events that endanger the collective health of populations living across geographical regions and international boundaries. As illustrated in this report, global health security, or lack of it, may also have an impact on economic or political stability, trade, tourism, access to goods and services and, if they occur repeatedly, on demographic stability. Global public health security embraces a wide range of complex and daunting issues, from the international stage to the individual household, including the health consequences of human behaviour, weather-related events and infectious diseases, and natural catastrophes and man-made disasters, all of which are discussed in this report.

The delicate balance between humans and microbes has been conditioned over generations of contact, exposure to immune systems and human behaviour. Today, it has shifted so that the equilibrium is driven by changes in human demographics and behaviour, economic development and land use, international travel and commerce, changing climate and ecosystems, poverty, conflict, famine and the deliberate release of infectious or chemical agents. This has heightened the risk of disease outbreaks.

chapter

1

It is estimated that 2.1 billion airline passengers travelled in 2006 (1). This means that diseases now have the potential to spread geographically much faster than at any time in history. An outbreak or epidemic in one part of the world is only a few hours away from becoming an imminent threat elsewhere.

Infectious diseases can not only spread faster, they appear to be emerging more quickly than ever before. Since the 1970s, new diseases have been identified at the unprecedented rate of one or more per year. There are now at least 40 diseases that were unknown a generation ago. In addition, during the last five years, WHO has verified more than 1100 epidemic events.

The lessons of history are a good starting point for this report as they exemplify the huge challenges to health that occur repeatedly and relentlessly. Some infectious diseases that have persisted for thousands of years still pose threats on a global scale.

BUILDING ON HISTORICAL LANDMARKS

Since they first walked the planet, human beings have struggled – and often failed – to protect themselves against adversaries that destroy their health, inhibit their ability to function and, ultimately, cause their death. It is only in relatively modern times that they have made lasting progress in preventing or controlling infectious diseases, as illustrated by three important historical landmarks in public health. While these advances are still of great relevance today, they need to be adapted and reinforced to confront the challenges to come.

Plague and quarantine

The practice of separating people with disease from the healthy population is an ancient one, with both biblical and Koranic references to the isolation of lepers. By the 7th century, China had a well-established policy of detaining sailors and foreign travellers suffering from plague.

The term "quarantine" dates from the late 14th century and the isolation of people arriving from plague-infected areas to the port of Ragusa, at the time under the control of the Venetian Republic. In 1397, the period was set at 40 days (the word quarantine being derived from the Italian for "forty"). Similar actions were taken by many other Mediterranean ports soon afterwards. Such public health measures became widespread and international over the following centuries, with committees often being appointed in cities to coordinate them (2). Figure 1.1 shows the rapid spread of bubonic plague across Europe in the mid-14th century.

The continuing devastation regularly wrought by plague and other epidemic diseases demonstrated that crude quarantine measures alone were largely ineffective. In the 17th century, an attempt to keep plague, which was spreading through continental Europe, from reaching England obliged all London-bound ships to wait at the mouth of the River Thames for at least 40 days. The attempt failed and plague caused devastation in England in 1665 and 1666. During the 18th century, all major towns and cities along the eastern seaboard of the United States passed quarantine laws, which typically were enforced only when epidemics seemed imminent.

In recent years, the most serious outbreak of plague occurred in five states in India in 1994, where almost 700 suspected bubonic or pneumonic plague cases and 56 deaths were reported to WHO, as required by the International Health Regulations (1969). The outbreak, which captured international media attention, resulted in catastrophic

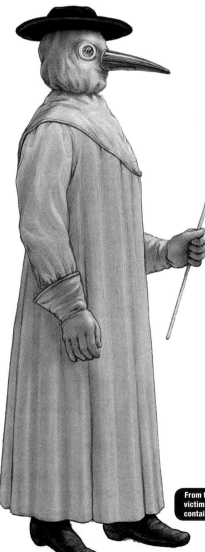

From the 14th century, European doctors visiting plague victims wore protective clothing, a mask and a beak containing strong-smelling herbs.

Figure 1.1 Spread of bubonic plague in Europe

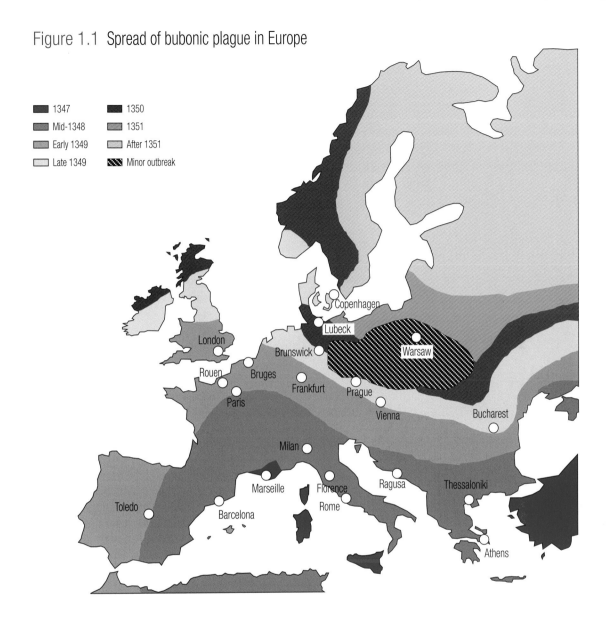

- 1347
- Mid-1348
- Early 1349
- Late 1349
- 1350
- 1351
- After 1351
- Minor outbreak

economic consequences for India when a number of countries overstepped the measures set out in IHR (1969) and imposed unnecessary travel and trade restrictions. The outbreak was brought under control within two months. During that period, more than 2 million tourism-related trips to the country were estimated to have been cancelled. Overall, the reported outbreak cost India approximately US$ 1.7 billion in lost trade and travel and caused a record trade deficit in 1994 (3). Since then, there have been many smaller, unrelated bubonic plague outbreaks in countries such as Algeria, the Democratic Republic of the Congo, Malawi and Zambia.

Cholera and sanitation

As with virtually all scientific advances, the physician John Snow's famous work on cholera – notably during the 1854 epidemic in London – did not emerge from a vacuum but was based on years of careful recording of outbreaks and heated debate as to the causes. Snow observed of cholera in 1855, "It travels along the great tracks of human intercourse, never going faster than people travel, and generally much more slowly. In extending to a fresh island or continent, it always appears first at a seaport. It never attacks the crews of ships going from a country free from cholera, to one where the disease is prevailing, till they have entered a port" (4).

During the London epidemic, Snow mapped the locations of homes of those who had died and noted that, in the Broad Street area, cases were clustered around a particular water pump. There was an underground sewer running close to the well, and people had reported the water from the well to be foul smelling in the days before the outbreak. As soon as Snow persuaded the authorities to remove the pump handle, the number of cases and deaths from cholera fell rapidly.

While the role of the pump handle removal in the decreased mortality rate has been debated, Snow's demonstration that cholera was associated with water was a powerful rebuttal of "miasma" theories of transmission through poisonous vapours. His work eventually led to improvements in sanitation in the United Kingdom that reduced the threat of cholera – though not to the same extent as endemic diarrhoeal disease from other causes (5). A new sewage system was constructed in London in the 1880s.

Cholera continues to be a major health risk all over the world. Latin America had been free of it for more than a century until, in 1991, a pandemic that had begun 30 years earlier and spread throughout many countries in Africa, Asia and Europe struck with devastating human and economic consequences. Thought to have originated from seafood contaminated by the bilge of ships off the coast of Peru, the disease spread rapidly across the continent and resulted in nearly 400 000 reported cases and over 4000 deaths in 16 countries that year. By 1995, there were more than 1 million cases and just over 10 000 deaths reported in the WHO Region of the Americas (6). In addition to human suffering and death, the outbreak provoked panic, disrupted social and economic structures, threatened development in affected populations, and led to extreme and unnecessary international reactions (7). Some neighbouring countries imposed trade and travel restrictions on Peru, as did European Union countries, the United States and others. Losses from trade embargoes, damage to tourism, and lost production attributable to cholera-related illnesses and death were estimated to be as much as US$ 1.5 billion (8).

The need to provide sanitation both for drinking-water and hygiene remains a huge challenge today in developing countries. Currently 1.1 billion people lack access to safe water and 2.6 billion people lack access to proper sanitation. As a result, more than 4500 children under five years of age die every day from easily preventable diseases such as diarrhoea. Many others, including older children and adults, especially women, suffer from poor health, diminished productivity and missed opportunities for education.

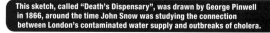

This sketch, called "Death's Dispensary", was drawn by George Pinwell in 1866, around the time John Snow was studying the connection between London's contaminated water supply and outbreaks of cholera.

Smallpox and immunization

Smallpox is one of the oldest known human diseases. There is evidence of its existence over 3000 years ago in Egypt: the mummified head of Ramses V, who died in 1157 BC, shows a pustular eruption that may have been caused by smallpox. It may have existed in parts of Asia about the same time and appears to have been introduced into China about the year 50 AD, to parts of Europe in the following few centuries, to western Africa in the 10th century, and to the Americas in the 16th century during the Spanish conquests.

During the 18th century, smallpox killed every seventh child born in Russia and every 10th child born in France and Sweden. Edward Jenner's experiment in 1796 brought hope that the disease could be controlled. Jenner, an English physician, realized that many of his patients who had been exposed to cowpox, the much milder but related disease, were immune to smallpox. He inoculated an eight-year-old farm boy with cowpox virus and, after observing the reaction, reinoculated him with smallpox virus. The boy did not develop the deadly disease, demonstrating that inoculation with cowpox could protect against smallpox. Jenner's procedure was soon widely accepted, resulting in sharp falls in smallpox death rates.

At the beginning of the 20th century, smallpox was still endemic in almost every country in the world. In the early 1950s, an estimated 50 million cases occurred globally each year with an estimated 15 million deaths, figures which fell to around 10–15 million cases and 3 million deaths by 1967 as access to immunizations increased.

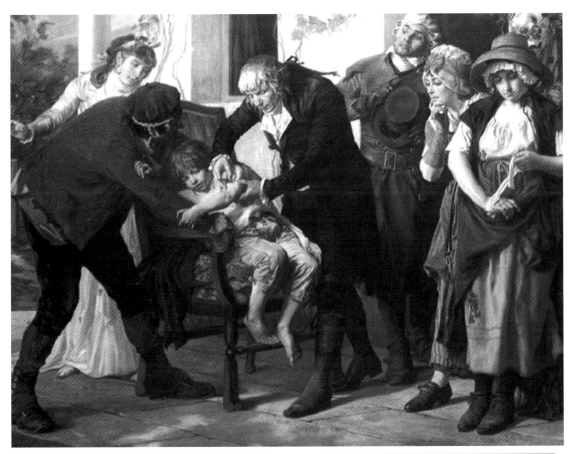

An English doctor, Edward Jenner, carries out the first vaccination against smallpox in 1796 by inoculating a boy with cowpox virus.

6

world health report 2007
global public health security
in the 21st century

Through the success of the 10-year global eradication campaign that began in 1967, the global eradication of smallpox was certified in 1979 (*9*).

Since eradication was certified, allegations have been made that some countries and terrorist groups may be storing smallpox virus, and its potential as a bioterrorist threat is causing major concern in many industrialized countries (*10*). Work is under way on a new and safer vaccine against smallpox, which would need to be produced in huge quantities if immunization against a deliberate release were to be undertaken.

Almost 30 years after its successful eradication, smallpox has, therefore, become a significant public health concern in terms of the deliberate release of the virus to cause harm. According to a recent WHO report, "the greatest fear is that in the absence of global capacity to contain an outbreak rapidly, smallpox might re-establish endemicity, undoing one of public health's greatest achievements" (*10*).

FOSTERING INTERNATIONAL COOPERATION

The three advances described above – in quarantine, sanitation and immunization – came about separately but gradually came to be seen as requiring international coordination in order to strengthen global public health security (see Box 1.1).

By the end of the 19th century, dozens of international conferences on disease control had been held, ultimately leading to the foundation of WHO in 1948 and the promulgation of the International Sanitary Regulations in 1951 (see Box 1.2).

The reasons for such international action were clear. One hundred years ago, infectious diseases such as cholera, plague and yellow fever – and many more such as diarrhoeal diseases other than cholera, influenza, malaria, pneumonias and tuberculosis – ravaged most civilizations and threatened public health security. They dominated entire regions and at times spread in pandemics across the globe. With few exceptions, there was little that could be done to halt their progression, until spectacular advances in medicine and public health during the first half of the 20th century yielded new drugs and vaccines that could prevent or cure infections. These advances helped industrialized countries, which had reliable access to them, to eliminate or markedly decrease the infectious disease threats. At the same time, improvements in hygiene and standards of living in these more prosperous parts of the world altered the conditions that had allowed the diseases to flourish.

While it can be argued that the means currently exist to prevent, control or treat most infectious diseases, paradoxically, the continuing likelihood of pandemics is still a huge threat to public health security, principally for two reasons. First, some of these diseases continue to thrive in developing countries where the ability to detect and respond is limited, leading to the potential for them to spread internationally at great speed. Second, new diseases emerging in human populations on a sporadic basis are often the result of a breach in the species barrier between humans and animals, permitting microbes that infect animals to infect humans as well, causing unexpected outbreaks that can also spread internationally. Therefore, international measures to prevent the spread of infectious diseases continue to remain essential in the 21st century.

Box 1.2 International collaboration on infectious disease control

Timeline of significant events in public health

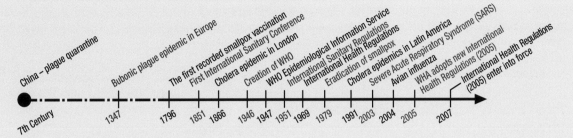

Largely provoked by the cholera pandemic of the time, threats of plague and the ineffectiveness of quarantine measures, many European leaders of the mid-19th century began to recognize that controlling the spread of infectious diseases from one nation to another required that they cooperate. International conventions were organized and draft covenants signed, almost all of which related to quarantine regulations (*8*).

From 1851 to 1900, 10 International Sanitary Conferences were convened, comprising a group of about 12 European countries or states, and focusing exclusively on the containment of epidemics within their territories. The inaugural 1851 conference in Paris lasted six months and established the vital principle that health protection was a proper subject for international consultations.

During the 1880s, a small group of South American nations signed the first set of international public health agreements in the Americas. In addition to cholera and plague, often carried among the huge numbers of immigrants arriving from Europe, these agreements covered yellow fever, which was endemic in much of the region. In 1892, the first International Sanitary Convention dealing only with cholera was signed. Five years later, at the 10th International Sanitary Conference, a similar convention focusing on plague was also signed. Important new policies emerged, such as the obligatory telegraphic notification of first cases of cholera and plague.

In 1902, 12 countries attended the First International Sanitary Convention of the American Republics in Washington, DC, the United States, leading to the creation of the Pan American Sanitary Bureau (now called the Pan American Health Organization). Its counterpart in Europe,

the Office International d'Hygiène Publique (OIHP), was established in 1907 and based in Paris (*11*).

Apart from its immediate toll on human lives, the First World War brought in its wake many epidemics resulting from the destruction of public health infrastructure, from typhus in Russia that threatened to spread to western Europe, to cholera, smallpox, dysentery and typhoid in the Ottoman Empire. These epidemics were the basis for the formation of the League of Nations Health Organisation, itself stemming from the newly created League of Nations. In 1920, the Health Organisation set up a temporary epidemic commission whose task was to help direct work in afflicted countries.

In 1951, three years after its founding, WHO adopted a revised version of the International Sanitary Regulations first approved in 1892. They focused on the control of cholera, plague, smallpox, typhoid fever and yellow fever. Their approach was still rooted in misunderstandings of the 19th century – that certain measures at border posts could alone prevent the spread of infectious diseases across international borders. They were succeded by IHR (1969), which required Member States to report outbreaks of certain diseases. Recent events have demonstrated the urgent need for a revised set of regulations with broader disease coverage, and measures to stop their spread across borders based on real time epidemiological evidence rather than pre-determined measures concentrated at borders. The IHR (2005) respond to this need and have now come into force (*12*).

8

world health report 2007
global public health security
in the 21st century

A new code for international health security

Ways of collectively working together in the face of emergency events of international health importance are reflected in the new revised International Health Regulations (2005). The Regulations, first issued in 1969, and discussed later in this chapter, were revised according to understanding and experience accumulated in the 1990s in response to changes in the human world, the microbial world, the natural environment and human behaviour, all of which posed increased threats to global public health security (these events are described in Chapter 2). An agreed code of conduct was required that could not only prevent and control such threats but could also provide a public health response to them while avoiding unnecessary interference with international trade and traffic.

The basis of an effective global system of epidemic alert and response was initiated by WHO in 1996. It was built essentially on a concept of international partnership with many other agencies and technical institutions. Systematic mechanisms for gathering epidemic intelligence and verifying the existence of outbreaks were established and prompted risk assessments, information dissemination and rapid field response. The Global Outbreak Alert and Response Network (GOARN) was set up as a technical partnership of existing institutions and networks to pool human and technical resources for the rapid identification, confirmation and response to outbreaks of international importance. The network provides an operational and coordination framework to access this expertise and skill, and to keep the international community constantly alert to the threat of outbreaks and ready to respond.

Coordinated by WHO, the network is made up of over 140 technical partners from more than 60 countries. These partners' institutions and networks provide rapid international multidisciplinary technical support for outbreak response. Figure 1.2 shows a sample of international epidemic response missions in the field in 1998 and 1999.

Figure 1.2 Examples of international epidemic response missions, 1998–1999

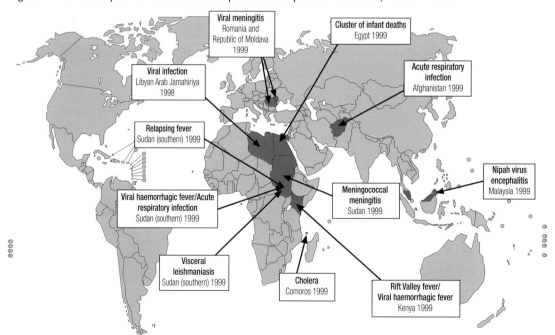

Between 2000 and 2005, there were more than 70 GOARN international outbreak responses, involving over 500 experts in the field. Regional and global mechanisms for stockpiling and rapid distribution of vaccines, drugs and specialized investigation and protection equipment have been established for haemorrhagic fevers, influenza, meningitis, smallpox and yellow fever. A specialized logistics response unit has been developed for epidemic response that allows WHO and its partners to be operational in extreme environments.

As part of ongoing efforts to improve operational coordination and information management, WHO is updating its event management system to support real time operational communications and access to critical information on epidemics. The Organization continues to strengthen specialized surveillance networks for dangerous pathogens, including dengue, influenza and plague.

In addition, the unique, large-scale active surveillance network developed by the Global Polio Eradication Initiative is being used to support surveillance of many other vaccine-preventable diseases, such as measles, meningitis, neonatal tetanus and yellow fever. This network is also regularly supporting outbreak surveillance and response activities for other health emergencies and outbreaks, including avian influenza, Ebola, Marburg haemorrhagic fever, SARS and yellow fever.

With its local knowledge of communities, health systems and government structures, the polio network has the technical capacity to plan and monitor immunization campaigns, during which the health officers are often the community's first point of entry into the health system for a range of diseases and conditions. The polio network is also called upon during outbreaks of meningitis and yellow fever and often helps to sustain international and national relief efforts, such as during the responses to the South-East Asia tsunami in December 2004 and the Pakistan earthquake in October 2005. Once polio eradication has been completed, continued investment in this network to broaden the skills of surveillance officers, immunization staff and laboratories, will increase capacity nationally and internationally for surveillance and response of vaccine-preventable and other outbreak-prone infectious diseases.

At the national level, collaboration between donor and recipient countries, which focuses on ensuring the technical and other resources to meet national core needs in disease detection and response, is a crucial factor in building the capacity to further strengthen global public health security. Effective implementation requires countries to invest in, manage and improve the functioning of a number of public health system components. These include epidemiological surveillance and information management systems, public health laboratory facilities, health and preparedness planning, health communication and intersectoral collaboration.

In order to ensure the maximum possible global public health security, countries – in collaboration with WHO and other relevant international organizations – must develop, maintain and strengthen appropriate public health and administrative capacities in general, not only at international ports, airports and land crossings. This requires close collaboration not only between WHO offices and Member States, but also among Member States themselves. Such multilateral cooperation will better prepare the world for future public health emergencies.

10

world health report 2007
global public health security
in the 21st century

International preparedness for chemical emergencies

It has long been recognized that many countries have limited capacities to detect and respond to chemical incidents, and that such events occurring in one country could have an impact on others. Equally recognized has been the need to strengthen both national and global public health preparedness and response. World Health Assembly resolution WHA55.16 (*13*) urges Member States to strengthen systems for surveillance, emergency preparedness and response for the release of chemical and biological agents and radionuclear materials in order to mitigate the potentially serious global public health consequences of such releases (see Chapter 2).

In 2002, WHO established the Chemical Incident Alert and Response System to operate along similar lines to the alert and response system for communicable diseases. In 2006, this system was extended to cover other environmental health emergencies, including those related to the disruption of environmental health services, such as water supply and sanitation, as well as radiological events.

An integral part of the system is ChemiNet, which pools human and technical resources for detecting, verifying and responding to environmental health events of (potential) international public health concern. ChemiNet draws on human and technical resources from institutions, agencies and academia in Member States as well as from international organizations, as illustrated in Figure 1.3.

ChemiNet is designed to mitigate chemical incidents and outbreaks of illness of chemical etiology that are of international public health concern by early detection, assessment and verification of outbreaks; provision of rapid, appropriate and effective assistance in response to outbreaks; and contribution to long-term preparedness and capacity building – the same protocol utilized in response to any public health emergency. In accordance with IHR (2005), ChemiNet provides a source of intelligence by informing WHO of chemical incidents or outbreaks of illness of potential international public health importance.

Prevention of and preparedness for uncontrolled chemical releases are part of a continuum of activities in ChemiNet that also encompass event detection, response and recovery. Since large-scale chemical incidents, such as that in Bhopal, India (see Chapter 2), shocked the world, much has been learned about measures for prevention and preparedness concerning such occurrences. Even in technically advanced, well-resourced countries, however, the risks of a large-scale chemical release

Figure 1.3 International public health security: a global network of national health systems and technical partners, coordinated by WHO, founded on four major areas of work

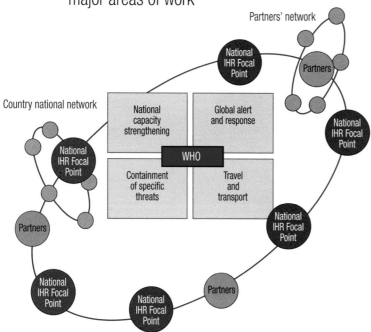

remain, particularly with the more recent threat of deliberate chemical release. No country can afford to be complacent.

Preventive measures include good land-use planning and enforcement so that chemical installations are not built close to places of high population density, the enforcement of high safety standards in chemical industries, and the monitoring of food, water and air quality to detect chemical contamination.

Preparedness measures include ensuring that there is a well-designed and rehearsed chemical emergency plan in place that involves all stakeholders, that local health-care facilities are informed about chemical risks in their catchment area, and that they are provided with the necessary decontamination and medical equipment. National capacity for detection of outbreaks caused by chemical releases includes the availability of a 24-hour poisons centre. Some countries, such as the United States, have fully integrated poison centres into their public health surveillance systems.

Since chemicals released into the environment can spread beyond the immediate vicinity of the event and, in some cases, have the potential to cross national borders, there is also a need for coordination of international preparedness and response. Some international agreements already exist, such as the United Nations Economic Commission for Europe (UNECE) Convention on the Transboundary Effects of Industrial Accidents (*14*).

The International Health Regulations (2005) and World Health Assembly resolution WHA55.16 (*13*) provide a framework for preparedness. Within this framework, WHO can conduct activities to respond immediately to events that threaten global public health security and can work collectively and proactively to prepare for such events. Chapter 4 shows how the framework can be applied to the current threats of avian influenza, XDR-TB and natural disasters.

New health regulations in a vastly altered world
As outlined earlier, concern about the international spread of infectious disease outbreaks and other events that threaten global public health security is not a modern phenomenon. In the past, attempts have often been made to stop these events from spreading by enforcing border controls. In the globalized world of the 21st century, although there is still collective interest in preventing the international spread of diseases, it is understood that borders alone cannot accomplish this. In recent decades, diseases have spread faster than ever before, aided by high-speed travel and the trade in goods and services between countries and continents, often during the incubation period before the signs and symptoms of disease are visible. The rapid spread of disease can only be prevented if there is immediate alert and response to disease outbreaks and other incidents that could spark epidemics or spread globally and if there are national systems in place for detection and response should such events occur across international borders. GOARN and ChemiNet are examples of such systems.

The aim of the collaboration set out in IHR (1969) was to achieve maximum protection against the international spread of disease with minimal disruption to trade and travel. Based mainly on attempts to stop the spread of disease through control measures at international borders, IHR (1969) offered a legal framework for the notification of and response to six diseases – cholera, plague, relapsing fever, smallpox, typhus and yellow fever – but suffered from very patchy compliance among WHO Member States.

From 1996 to 2005, Member States examined and revised IHR (1969) in order to meet the new challenges that had arisen in the control of emerging and re-emerging infectious diseases, including the rapid global transit of diseases and the exchange of animals and goods that may inadvertently carry infectious agents. Several emerging and re-emerging diseases identified in this period are shown in Figure 1.4. Another challenge was the management of near instantaneous modes of communication, such as mobile telephones and the Internet, which have the potential to cause panic in populations. The resulting revised Regulations – IHR (2005) (*12*) – came into force in June 2007. They provide a legal framework for reporting significant public health risks and events that are identified within national boundaries and for the recommendation of context-specific measures to stop their international spread, rather than establishing pre-determined measures aimed at stopping diseases at international borders as in the case of IHR (1969).

The IHR (2005) define an emergency as an "extraordinary event" that could spread internationally or might require a coordinated international response. Events that may constitute a public health emergency of international concern are assessed by State Parties using a decision instrument and, if particular criteria are met, WHO must be notified (see chapter 5). Mandatory notification is called for in a single case of a disease that could threaten global public health security: smallpox, poliomyelitis caused by a wild-type poliovirus, human influenza caused by a new virus subtype, and SARS. In parallel, a second limited list includes diseases of documented – but

Figure 1.4 Selected emerging and re-emerging infectious diseases: 1996–2004

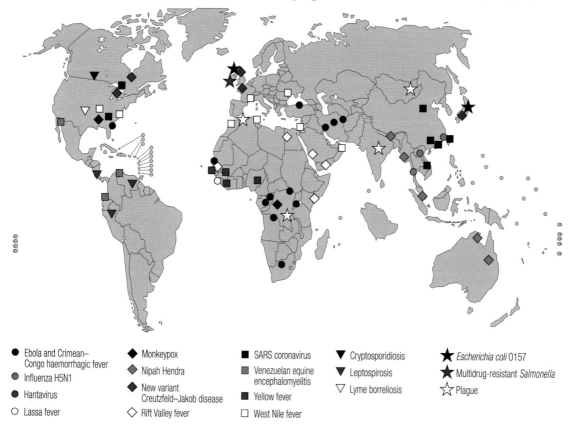

- ● Ebola and Crimean–Congo haemorrhagic fever
- ● Influenza H5N1
- ● Hantavirus
- ○ Lassa fever
- ◆ Monkeypox
- ◆ Nipah Hendra
- ◆ New variant Creutzfeld–Jakob disease
- ◇ Rift Valley fever
- ■ SARS coronavirus
- ■ Venezuelan equine encephalomyelitis
- ■ Yellow fever
- □ West Nile fever
- ▼ Cryptosporidiosis
- ▼ Leptospirosis
- ▽ Lyme borreliosis
- ★ *Escherichia coli* O157
- ★ Multidrug-resistant *Salmonella*
- ☆ Plague

not inevitable – international impact. An event involving a disease on this second list, which includes cholera, pneumonic plague, yellow fever, viral haemorrhagic fevers (Ebola, Lassa and Marburg), West Nile fever and other diseases that are of national or regional concern, should always result in the use of the decision instrument of the Regulations that permits evaluation of the risk of international spread. Thus, the two safeguards create a baseline of security by obliging countries to respond in designated ways to well-known threats.

The broad definitions of "public health emergency of international concern" and "disease" allow for the inclusion in IHR (2005) of threats beyond infectious diseases, including those caused by the accidental or intentional release of pathogens or chemical or radionuclear materials. The basic epidemiological, laboratory and investigative principles, and the verification and notification procedures, are fundamentally the same for all events. Moreover, such events are routinely included in the daily global surveillance activities undertaken by WHO through many different networks of collaborating laboratories and surveillance networks. Many of these events are automatically picked up by the Global Public Health Intelligence Network (GPHIN) (15), an electronic intelligence-gathering tool, thus providing a safety net for detection of events not otherwise reported. The inclusion of public health emergencies other than infectious diseases extends the scope of the Regulations to protect global public health security in a comprehensive way.

The IHR (2005) redirect the focus from an almost exclusive concentration on measures at seaports and airports aimed at blocking the importation of cases towards a rapid response at the source of an outbreak. They introduce a set of "core capacity requirements" that all countries must meet in order to detect, assess, notify and report the events covered by the Regulations. Rather than take to task violators, the new Regulations aim to strengthen collaboration on a global scale by seeking to improve capacity and demonstrate to countries that compliance is in their best interests. Thus, compliance has three compelling incentives: to reduce the disruptive consequences of an outbreak, to speed its containment and to maintain good standing in the eyes of the international community. Collaboration between Member States, especially between developed and developing countries, to ensure the availability of technical and other resources is a crucial factor not only in implementing the Regulations, but also in building and strengthening public health capacity and the networks and systems that strengthen global public health security.

A revolutionary departure from previous international conventions and regulations is the fact that IHR (2005) explicitly acknowledge that non-state sources of information about outbreaks will often pre-empt official notifications. This includes situations where countries may be reluctant to reveal an event in their territories. WHO is now authorized through IHR (2005) to take into account information sources other than official notifications. WHO will always seek verification of such information from the country involved before taking any action on it. This reflects yet another of the realities stemming from the SARS outbreak: in an electronically transparent world where outbreaks are particularly newsworthy events, their concealment is no longer a viable option for governments. Also, at a time when information is shared at the click of a button, reputable sources of information are critical in maintaining public awareness and support of prevention and control measures.

The sudden emergence in 2003 of SARS was a vivid example of how an infectious disease can pose a serious threat to global public health security, the livelihood of populations, the functioning of health systems and the stability and growth of economies.

The major lessons learned from SARS and other diseases, discussed in Chapter 3, have been not only the need to collectively build up surveillance and information systems that enable timely reporting and response, but also the need to improve infection control capacity. Unfortunately, these capabilities are often lacking and so vulnerability to acute public health events will not simply go away. They need to be confronted urgently. The question is: how can this best be done?

Part of the answer relates to the background factors or causes that lead or contribute to epidemics and other acute health emergencies. These may be natural, environmental, industrial, human, accidental or deliberate. Some of the most important of these causes, and examples of their recent impact in different parts of the world, are discussed in the next chapter.

REFERENCES

1. *Fact sheet: IATA*. Geneva, International Air Transport Association, 2007 (http://www.iata.org/pressroom/facts_figures/fact_sheets/iata.htm, accessed 10 May 2007).
2. Porter R. *The greatest benefit to mankind: a medical history of humanity, from antiquity to the present*. London, Harper Collins, 1997.
3. International notes update: human plague, India, 1994. *Morbidity and Mortality Weekly Report*, 1994, 43:761–762 (http://www.cdc.gov/mmwr/preview/mmwrhtml/00032992.htm, accessed 11 April 2007).
4. Davey Smith G. Behind the Broad Street pump: aetiology, epidemiology and prevention of cholera in mid-19th century Britain [commentary]. *International Journal of Epidemiology*, 2003, 31:920–932.
5. Cairncross S. Water supply and sanitation: some misconceptions [editorial]. *Tropical Medicine and International Health*, 2003, 8:193–195.
6. Cholera in the Americas. *Epidemiological Bulletin of the Pan American Health Organization,* 1995, 16(2) (http://www.paho.org/english/sha/epibul_95-98/be952choleraam.htm, accessed 11 April 2007).
7. *Global epidemics and impact of cholera*. Geneva, World Health Organization (http://www.who.int/topics/cholera/impact/en/index.html, accessed 11 April 2007).
8. Knobler S, Mahmoud A, Lemon S, Pray L, eds. *The impact of globalization on infectious disease emergence and control: exploring the consequences and opportunities. Workshop summary – Forum on Microbial Threats.* Washington, DC, The National Academies Press, 2006.
9. Fenner F, Henderson DA, Arita I, Jezek Z, Ladnyi ID. *Smallpox and its eradication*. Geneva, World Health Organization, 1988.
10. *Global smallpox vaccine reserve: report by the Secretariat*. Geneva, World Health Organization, 2005 (report to the WHO Executive Board, document EB115/36; http://www.who.int/gb/ebwha/pdf_files/EB115/B115_36-en.pdf, accessed 11 May 2007).
11. Howard-Jones N. *The scientific background of the International Sanitary Conferences 1851–1938*. Geneva, World Health Organization, 1975.
12. *International Health Regulations (2005)*. Geneva, World Health Organization, 2006 (http://www.who.int/csr/ihr/en/, accessed 18 April 2007).
13. *Global public health response to natural occurrence, accidental release or deliberate use of biological and chemical agents or radionuclear material that affect health*. Geneva, World Health Organization, 2002 (World Health Assembly resolution WHA55.16; http://www.who.int/gb/ebwha/pdf_files/WHA55/ewha5516.pdf, accessed 13 May 2007).
14. Convention on the transboundary effects of industrial accidents. Geneva, United Nations Economic Commission for Europe, 1992 (http://www.unece.org/env/teia/welcome.htm, accessed 14 May 2007).
15. *Information: Global Public Health Intelligence Network (GPHIN)*. Ottawa, Public Health Agency of Canada, 2004 (http://www.phac-aspc.gc.ca/media/nr-rp/2004/2004_gphin-rmispbk_e.html, accessed 3 May 2007).

THREATS
TO PUBLIC HEALTH
SECURITY

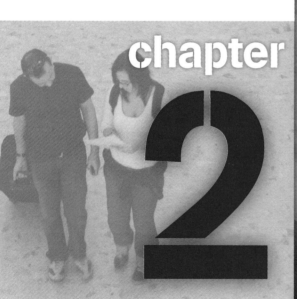

chapter

2

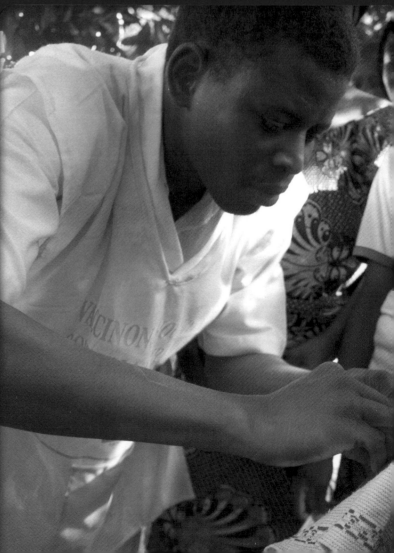

Chapter 2 explores a range of threats to global public health security, as defined by the International Health Regulations (2005), which result from human actions or causes, from human interaction with the environment, and from sudden chemical and radioactive events, including industrial accidents and natural phenomena. It begins by illustrating how inadequate investment in public health, resulting from a false sense of security in the absence of infectious disease outbreaks, has led to reduced vigilance and a relaxing of adherence to effective prevention programmes.

The new regulations are no longer limited to the scope of their original six diseases – cholera, plague, relapsing fever, smallpox, typhus and yellow fever. Rather, they address "illness or medical conditions, irrespective of origin or source that present or could present significant harm to humans" (*1*).

Such threats to public health security, be they epidemics of infectious diseases, natural disasters, chemical emergencies or certain other acute health events, can be traced to one or more causes. The causes may be natural, environmental, industrial, accidental or deliberate but – more often than not – they are related to human behaviour.

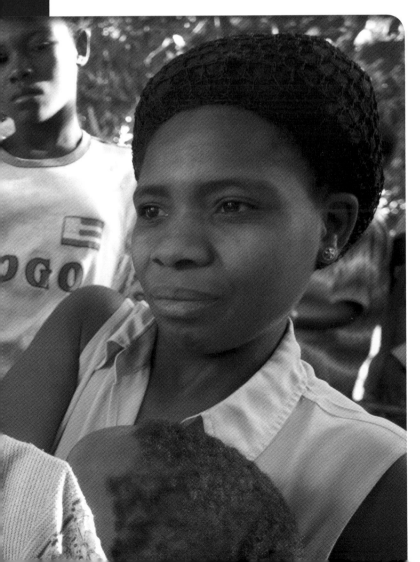

This chapter explores the threats to global public health security, as defined by IHR (2005), which can result from human action or inaction and natural events. The importance of the more fundamental causes of health security embedded in the social and political environments that foster inequities within and between groups of people will be discussed in subsequent publications.

HUMAN CAUSES OF PUBLIC HEALTH INSECURITY

Human behaviour that determines public health security includes decisions and actions taken by individuals at all levels – for example, political leaders, policy-makers, military commanders, public health specialists and the general population – which have dramatic health consequences, both negative and positive. The following examples illustrate the public health security repercussions when human behaviour is influenced by situations of conflict and displacement or attitudes of complacency, lack of commitment, and mistrust and misinformation.

Inadequate investment

Inadequate investment in public health, resulting from a false sense of security in the absence of infectious disease outbreaks, can lead to reduced vigilance and a relaxing of adherence to effective prevention programmes. For example, following the widespread use of insecticides in large-scale, systematic control programmes, by the late 1960s most of the important vector-borne diseases were no longer considered major public health problems outside of sub-Saharan Africa. Control programmes then lapsed as resources dwindled, and the training and employment of specialists declined. The result was that within the next 20 years, many important vector-borne diseases including African trypanosomiasis, dengue and dengue haemorrhagic fever, and malaria emerged in new areas or re-emerged in areas previously affected. Urbanization and increasing international trade and travel have contributed to rapid spread of dengue viruses and their vectors. Dengue caused an unprecedented pandemic in 1998, with 1.2 million cases reported to WHO from 56 countries. Since then, dengue epidemics have continued, affecting millions of people from Latin America to South-East Asia. Globally, the average annual number of cases reported to WHO has nearly doubled in each of the last four decades.

Inadequate surveillance results from a lack of commitment to build effective health systems capable of monitoring a country's health status. This is illustrated by the rapid global emergence and spread of HIV/AIDS in the 1970s. The presence of a new health threat was not detected by what were invariably weak health systems in many developing countries, and only belatedly became a matter of international concern when it manifested itself in the first cases in the United States. Figure 2.1 shows developments over 25 years dating from this event at the beginning of the 1980s.

Surveillance is the cornerstone of public health security. Without appropriately designed and functioning surveillance systems, unusual but identifiable health events cannot be detected, monitored for their likely impact, quantified over time or measured for the effectiveness of interventions put in place to counteract them (see Figure 2.2).

The inability of surveillance systems to recognize new disease trends is not confined to poorer countries. For instance, the first cases of AIDS were detected and characterized in the United States not by surveillance but by serendipity. Epidemiologists at the United States Centers for Disease Control and Prevention (CDC) observed an unusual number of requests to their orphan drug repository for antimicrobials to treat pneumonia

Figure 2.1 Twenty-five years of HIV/AIDS

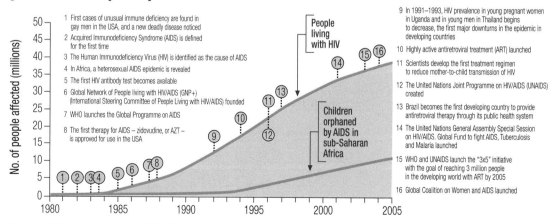

Source: *2006 Report on the global AIDS epidemic.* Geneva, Joint United Nations Programme on HIV/AIDS, 2006.

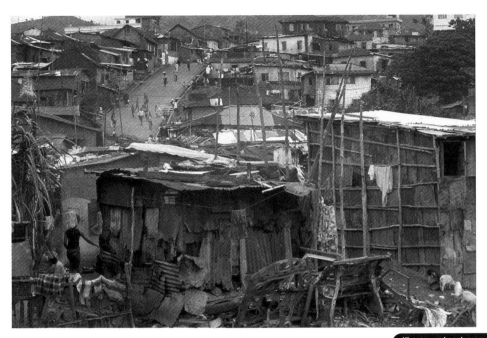

Viruses, such as dengue, flourish in slums that result from uncontrolled urbanization.

caused by *Pneumocystis carinii*, a rare parasitic infection but one that is common in AIDS cases (*2*). Yet, what soon became known as AIDS had been occurring for perhaps many years in Africa and Haiti – poorly detected and poorly characterized. Inadequate surveillance systems, universal in low and middle income countries, are not capable of recognizing unusual health events. Similarly, because these systems are poorly funded and diagnostic facilities are limited, the systems do not allow for the identification and monitoring of any but a few specific illnesses, for example, tuberculous. Ministries of health are doubly compromised because, without better surveillance, it is difficult for them to mount interventions or measure their effectiveness.

In addition to limited disease surveillance capacity and data, early efforts to control the AIDS epidemic were also hampered by a lack of solid data on sexual behaviour, whether in Africa, Haiti, or the United States and other industrialized countries. In the

Figure 2.2 Global outbreaks, the challenge: late reporting and response

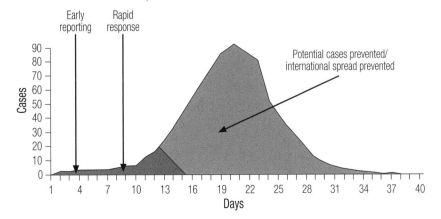

20

world health report 2007
global public health security
in the 21st century

industrialized world, the 1960s was a period of scientific advances and rapid social change. The widespread availability of oral contraception contributed to the apparent liberalization of sexual mores that was furthered by the profound social changes of that period. Coupled with these developments, attitudes towards and among homosexually active men became more liberal, particularly in the big cities of the United States, with a marked migration of gay men to certain key cities. Despite these significant social and attitudinal changes, no scientific study of sexual behaviour, and its relationship to the emergence of sexually transmitted diseases, had been carried out in the United States since the 1950s, and these were long out of date by the time AIDS appeared as a major public health threat.

As inadequate as behavioural data were in the industrialized world, they were practically non-existent in the developing world. The understanding of HIV/AIDS in the context of sexuality in the developing world took years to develop and is still poorly understood. Only in recent years, a quarter of a century after the description of AIDS, have population-based surveys of sexual behaviour (demographic and health surveys) been conducted that allow a better understanding – supported by valid scientific evidence – of sexual behaviour in countries on multiple continents heavily affected by HIV/AIDS (*3*).

Against a background of armed conflict, families have less access to health care and are more vulnerable to disease.

Unexpected policy changes

Even with reliable operations in place, unexpected policy changes in public health systems can have lethal and costly repercussions. Such was the case in August 2003, when unsubstantiated claims originating in northern Nigeria that the oral polio vaccine (OPV) was unsafe and could sterilize young children led to governments ordering the suspension of polio immunization in two northern states and substantial reductions in polio immunization coverage in a number of others. The result was a large outbreak of poliomyelitis across northern Nigeria and the reinfection of previously polio-free areas in the south of the country. This outbreak eventually paralysed thousands of children in Nigeria. The disease also spread from northern Nigeria to polio-free countries.

At the beginning of 2003, only seven countries in the world remained infected: Afghanistan, Egypt, India, Niger, Nigeria, Pakistan and Somalia. By the end of 2006, 19 polio-free countries in Africa, Asia and the Middle East had experienced outbreaks traceable genetically to the Nigerian virus. Mass outbreak response activities across these countries cost more than US$ 450 million. In July 2004, polio immunization resumed throughout northern Nigeria, as a result of a tremendous collaborative effort between state and federal authorities and traditional and religious leaders, supported by the high-level engagement of organizations such as the African Union and the Organization of the Islamic Conference – thus showing that collaboration and partnership that extend beyond the traditional discipline of health can bring tremendous change for the good of global public health security.

Public health consequences of conflict

When governments or armed groups engage in armed conflict, a collateral impact is often the destruction or weakening of health systems, resulting in their diminished capacity to detect, prevent and respond to infectious disease outbreaks, which in turn reduces the concerned population's access to health care. Such was the case in Angola. One consequence of the 27-year civil war (1975–2002) was the spread of an outbreak of Marburg haemorrhagic fever in 2004–2005, which affected more than 200 people, 90% of whom died (see Box 2.1). Transmission of Marburg haemorrhagic fever, an infectious disease related to Ebola, is amplified in situations where poor health facilities are overcrowded and understaffed, and where lack of investment in hospitals and clinics results in sub-standard infection control.

Human population movements on a large scale as a result of war, conflict or natural catastrophes have been tragically common in recent years. The forced migration or displacement of large numbers of people often oblige them to live in crowded,

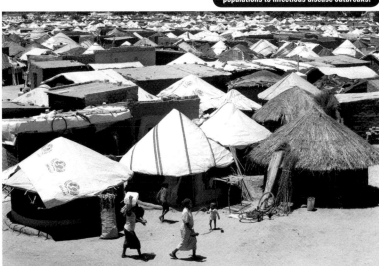

Overcrowding exposes displaced populations to infectious disease outbreaks.

unhygienic and impoverished conditions, which, in turn, heighten the risk of infectious disease epidemics. This was the cause of the cholera epidemic in the Democratic Republic of the Congo, in the aftermath of the crisis in Rwanda in 1994. In July of that year, between 500 000 and 800 000 people crossed the border to seek refuge in the outskirts of the Congolese city of Goma. During the first month after their arrival, close to 50 000 refugees died. The extremely high crude mortality rate of 20–35 per 10 000 per day can be associated with an explosive outbreak of combined cholera and shigella dysentery.

Box 2.1 Marburg haemorrhagic fever and health systems in conflict situations

Angola had witnessed almost three decades of conflict, which, apart from the immediate human casualties, had left the country with a severely damaged health infrastructure, a hospital system in dire need of basic equipment and supplies, inadequate communication and transport systems, and a population weakened by economic hardship. These weaknesses hampered efforts to contain the outbreak of Marburg haemorrhagic fever in 2005, as containment of an infectious disease depends on active surveillance mechanisms, the prompt detection and isolation of new cases in specially designated and equipped facilities, and the rapid tracing of contacts (4). The Angolan authorities, with the support of the international community, launched a massive effort to reconstruct health and transport systems and to improve the population's

nutrition. Despite their best attempts, 70% of the population is still without basic health care (5).

The outbreak of Marburg haemorrhagic fever in Angola was the largest on record, with the highest fatality rate, but it was not the only outbreak to occur following a conflict situation (6). Another large outbreak in the eastern region of the Democratic Republic of the Congo, made inaccessible by the conflict, occurred in late 1998. As many as 154 cases were reported, with 128 deaths. These were followed by sporadic cases with small chains of transmission over a two-year period. The war delayed access and evaluation, so that supplies were severely limited in all the health facilities in the region (7).

The speed of transmission and the high attack rate were related to the contamination with *Vibrio cholerae* of the only available source of water, Lake Kivu, and the absence of proper housing and sanitation (*8*).

The problems associated with people living in high density environments are not limited to emergency areas such as refugee camps. Rapid urbanization that has become common in many countries in the 21st century means that cities are now home to over half the world's population. Uncontrolled urbanization is characterized by expanding metropolitan areas, worsening environmental degradation, increasing inequity and the growth and proliferation of slums and informal settlements. Indeed, a third of global urban dwellers, or a billion people, live in slums and informal settlements where they exist in cramped, congested living conditions, without access to safe water, sanitation, safe food, decent shelter or meaningful employment.

Microbial evolution and antibiotic resistance

Another category of threats to public health security concerns the continuing and increasing evolution of resistance to anti-infective drugs, which is a major factor in the emergence and re-emergence of infectious diseases (*9*). Bacteria can develop resistance to antibiotics through spontaneous mutation and through the exchange of genes between strains and species of bacteria.

Bacteria often live in harmony with other inhabitants of the Earth. However, since penicillin became widely available in 1942, and other antibiotics soon followed, the killing and growth-inhibitory effects of antibiotics have applied selective pressure that has reduced the number of susceptible strains, leading to the propagation of more resistant varieties of bacteria (*10*). The selection and spread of these varieties are facilitated paradoxically by either over-prescribing or under-prescribing of drugs,

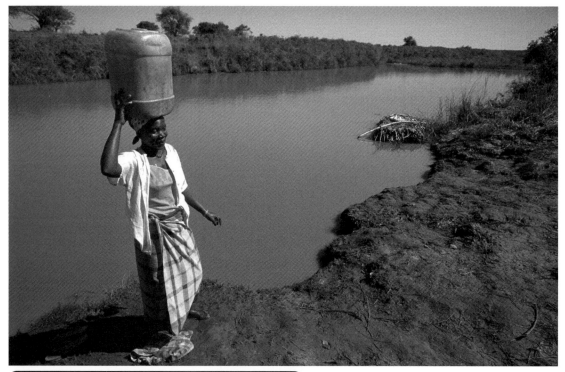

Contaminated lakes and rivers are often people's only sources of drinking-water.

poor compliance with recommended dosages, and unregulated sale by non-health workers (*9*). Antibiotics were initially developed for the treatment of infectious diseases in people, but eventually the same drugs also began to be used for the treatment of animals and plants. Often the same microbes circulate among their human, animal and agricultural hosts, providing opportunities for swapping or exchanging resistant genes and thus assisting the evolution and spread of resistance (*10*).

The discoverer of penicillin, Alexander Fleming, first warned of the potential importance of the development of resistance (*11*). Soon the evidence became alarming. In 1946, a hospital in the United Kingdom reported that 14% of all *Staphylococcus aureus* infections were resistant to penicillin. By 1950, this proportion had increased to 59%. In the 1990s, penicillin-resistant *S. aureus* had attained levels greater than 80% both in hospitals and in the community (see Figure 2.3).

It is not only bacteria that develop resistance to drugs: parasites do so too. By 1976, chloroquine-resistant *Plasmodium falciparum* malaria was highly prevalent in South-East Asia and 10 years later was found worldwide, as was high-level resistance to two back-up drugs, sulfadoxine pyrimethamine and mefloquine (*9*). The development of parasitic and bacterial resistance to drugs commonly used to treat malaria and tuberculosis is a grave threat to public health. The same is true for viruses, as shown by the emerging resistance to anti-HIV drugs (*9*).

Organisms that are resistant to multiple anti-infective drugs are not unusual (*12*). The results of resistance are very serious in terms of increased mortality, with a doubling of mortality being observed in some resistant infections as well as a need for an increase in the length of treatment with the more expensive anti-infective drugs or drug combinations. Complicating the matter, fewer new antibiotics are reaching the market with no new class of broad-spectrum antibiotic likely to appear soon. New public-private partnerships, however, are slowly beginning to fill the pipeline of new drugs for diseases such as tuberculosis and malaria, many of them with initial funding from the Bill and Melinda Gates Foundation (*9*).

The spread of resistance worldwide is one reason why efforts to detect and respond to outbreaks of infectious diseases as quickly as possible are so important, as is the wider need to rebuild and strengthen health systems, improve water and sanitation systems, minimize the impact of natural and human-influenced changes in the environment, effectively communicate information about the prevention of infectious diseases, and use anti-infective drugs appropriately (*9*). If the use of anti-infective drugs were better rationalized, the evolutionary pressure on bacteria would be altered and susceptible strains could again proliferate (*12*).

Figure 2.3 Evolution of penicillin resistance in *Staphylococcus aureus:* a continuing story

1928	Penicillin discovered
1942	Penicillin introduced
1945	Fleming warns of possible resistance
1946	14% hospital strains resistant
1950	59% hospital strains resistant
1960s–70s	Resistance spreads in communities
1980s–90s	Resistance exceeds 80% in communities, 95% in most hospitals

24

world health report 2007
global public health security
in the 21st century

Animal husbandry and food processing

Human spongiform encephalopathy

In May 1995, the death of a 19-year-old man in the United Kingdom marked the first human death of what is now known to be variant Creutzfeldt-Jakob disease (vCJD) or human bovine spongiform encephalopathy (BSE). His illness and death demonstrate the health consequences of improper animal rendering and feeding practices that had begun during the 10-year period prior to his death. Briefly, the carcasses of cattle, including those that had been infected with the BSE-causing agent, were rendered into livestock feed. Some of the cattle consuming this feed then also became infected leading to an epidemic of BSE, commonly called "mad cow disease" because of the animals' uncharacteristically agitated behaviour. From October 1996 to November 2002, 129 cases of vCJD were reported in the United Kingdom, six in France and one each in Canada, Ireland, Italy and the United States.

The most likely source of human infection with vCJD is the consumption of meat contaminated with BSE. The crisis, therefore, led to the recognition of the need for government intervention along the entire "feed to food" continuum to ensure the safety of foodstuffs for human consumption. Trade was shown to adapt itself very quickly to the changing regulatory environment, with immense consequences for the United Kingdom market.

Only reinforced surveillance in humans and animals can expose how widely the agent was exported during the late 1980s and mid-1990s from its original European focus and how far this public health security threat extends. The recent identification in the United Kingdom of a fourth case of vCJD associated with a blood transfusion that was later found to be contaminated with vCJD caused additional concern (13). This is a reminder of the need for adequate investment in ensuring as safe a blood supply as possible, taking into account risks of disease transmission in each country.

Nipah virus

Nipah virus is an emerging viral pathogen that causes encephalitis – an inflammation of the brain – which is fatal in up to 75% of the people that it infects. The disease caused by Nipah virus was first recognized in Peninsular Malaysia in an outbreak which began in September 1998 and ended in April 1999. During that outbreak, 265 human cases including 105 deaths were reported (14). When the reports of a severe encephalitis outbreak began to accumulate, it was initially attributed to Japanese encephalitis, a disease which is prevalent in Malaysia.

The belief that this outbreak was due to Japanese encephalitis resulted in expensive and disruptive campaigns directed at mass immunization and mosquito control. These control efforts were ineffective because it was in fact a new disease caused by a previously unrecognized virus.

The majority of human cases were associated with direct contact with sick or dying pigs or fresh pig products. It was eventually recognized that commercially raised pigs, often housed near fruit orchards, were acting as the intermediate hosts of the new virus. Transmission among pigs and from pigs to humans is now thought to have occurred via the aerosol route in the former or following contact with throat or nasal secretions in the latter. The end of the outbreak coincided with the mass culling of more than 1 million pigs, which was part of the control strategy. In Singapore, there was a small related outbreak that infected 11 human cases resulting in one death. A further 89 individuals were subsequently shown by serological tests to have experienced an asymptomatic or mild infection of the disease. The Singapore outbreak ended following a ban on the importation of pigs from Malaysia.

Evidence from additional Nipah virus outbreaks since the events in Malaysia and Singapore suggests that the virus may have become more pathogenic for humans. In these cases, it seems that the virus can spread to humans without an intermediate amplifying host such as the pig, and that human-to-human transmission can occur with even casual contact. Some evidence points to amplification of transmission within the health-care setting. In the most recent of these outbreaks, consumption of contaminated food is considered the most likely route of exposure for several human infections. Moreover, evidence of Nipah virus infection in fruit bats has now been found in a broader range of countries than previously assumed.

The emergence and subsequent evolution of Nipah virus illustrate many of the public health problems caused by emerging pathogens. These include initial diagnostic confusion leading to delayed detection and inappropriate control measures, and high mortality in the absence of effective preventive or control measures, which becomes more difficult when control of an intermediate host, such as the pig, is no longer an option. Changes in the epidemiological behaviour of the virus underscore the need to be ready to adapt control measures as a new pathogen evolves.

WEATHER-RELATED EVENTS AND INFECTIOUS DISEASES

Intensifying climatic conditions, together with a range of environmental, epidemiological and socioeconomic factors, are bringing about changes in the exposure of populations to infectious diseases, as illustrated by the following example of Rift Valley fever.

Above-normal rainfall associated with the occurrence of the warm phase of the El Niño Southern Oscillation phenomenon is increasing the breeding sites of mosquitoes, with a consequent rise in the number of outbreaks of Rift Valley fever. From December 1997 to March 1998, the largest outbreak ever reported in East Africa occurred in

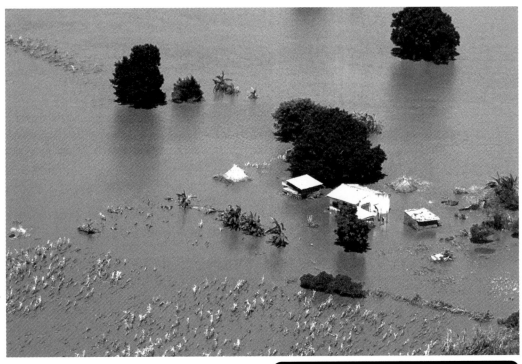

Above-normal rainfall increases the risk of vector-borne diseases.

Kenya, Somalia and the United Republic of Tanzania. The total number of human infections in the North Eastern Province of Kenya and southern Somalia alone was estimated at 89 000, with 478 "unexplained" deaths (*15*). Complications arising from Rift Valley fever in humans include retinopathy, blindness, meningo-encephalitis, haemorrhagic syndrome with jaundice, petechiae and death. The outbreaks in East Africa were linked to the higher than average rainfall – favouring the hatching of mosquito eggs – and a complex interaction between non-vaccinated cattle and the mosquitoes, which transmit the virus from animals to humans principally after feeding on infected animals. Female mosquitoes are also able to pass the infection to their offspring which spread the virus to animals on which they then feed, thus perpetuating a vicious circle of infection.

Animal immunization is only partially effective in preventing these outbreaks because it must be implemented prior to the beginning of an outbreak in animals and, if carried out during an outbreak, there is a risk of cross-infection from the reuse of needles and syringes.

After the 1997–1998 outbreaks, a new prevention strategy was developed based on two components: an accurate forecasting model, based on climatic conditions that can predict the emergence of Rift Valley fever 2–4 months in advance, and efficient veterinary public health services capable of implementing emergency mass animal immunization before the beginning of the animal outbreak.

Forecasting models and early warning systems for Rift Valley fever, based on satellite images and weather and climate forecasting data, were successfully developed to meet these requirements. In Africa and the Middle-East, collaboration with affected countries, space agencies (the United States National Aeronautics and Space Administration (NASA) and the International Reference Ionosphere (IRI) project), the Food and Agriculture Organization of the United Nations (FAO) and WHO made it possible to draw up a monthly map of the possible emergence zones for Rift Valley fever. These maps were used to inform the countries and help them with the early detection of cases. Ultimately, these forecasting alerts should allow authorities to implement measures to avert an impending epidemic by allowing implementation of mass animal immunization prior to the start of the animal outbreak and to conduct intensive social mobilization programmes aimed at changing risky behaviour.

On two occasions, the NASA/WHO monthly mapping of fever emergence was able to predict an animal outbreak one month before it surfaced. In November 2006, alert messages were sent to countries in the Horn of Africa. In addition, outbreaks of other arboviruses (dengue, West Nile fever and yellow fever) were reported in the at-risk areas for Rift Valley fever. These results show that the Rift Valley fever models may be useful for the forecasting and early detection of arbovirus outbreaks. Further progress is necessary in this area to refine models, but the use of predictive climatology for insect-borne diseases of animals should be encouraged.

While the precise impacts of epidemics are difficult to predict, the necessary public health response is clear. In such rapidly changing conditions, prevention is of the greatest importance; where prevention has failed, identifying and responding to epidemics becomes even more important.

OTHER PUBLIC HEALTH EMERGENCIES

The broad scope of the International Health Regulations (2005) allows for the inclusion of radionuclear and chemical events that have the potential to cause harm on a global scale. Such events, regardless of origin, rely on the same epidemiological principles of surveillance, early detection and response as biological threats in order to safeguard health.

Sudden chemical and radioactive events

For much of the world, life in the 21st century has become greatly dependent on chemical processing and nuclear power. Public health security in turn relies on the safety of these facilities and the appropriate use of their products. Major chemical spills, leaks and dumping, nuclear melt-downs, and the deliberate release of chemical or biological agents occupy yet another category of threats to public health security. The possibility of such events invokes the notion of surprise attack or accidents, innocent victims and malicious or negligent perpetrators, and causes fears that may be disproportionate to the real risk.

Most countries subscribe to international conventions banning chemical weapons. Incidents such as the release of sarin gas (the sole purpose of which is to harm the nervous system) on the Tokyo subway in 1995, however, remind us that although chemical and biological attacks are rare, there are individuals, groups and governments who are ready to use this brand of terrorism (see Box 2.2).

Similarly, chemical and nuclear processing plants operate under safety protocols, such as those outlined by the International Programme on Chemical Safety (*21*), to protect their workers, their facilities and the people and environment surrounding them. Nonetheless, human and mechanical errors occur and accidents happen, sometimes with devastating effects.

Wide-scale attacks using chemical weapons or major industrial accidents are not the full picture when it comes to the disease burden from chemical incidents. The majority of such deaths and illness is attributable to the many medium-sized and small-scale chemical incidents that take place every year around the world. Nevertheless,

---

Box 2.2 The deliberate use of chemical and biological agents to cause harm

Chemicals

The deliberate large-scale use of chemicals as poison gas weapons dates back to the First World War, when tear gas, mustard gas and phosgene were employed against troops in the trenches of European battlefields to deadly and disabling effect. Estimates range from about 1.17 to 1.25 million gas casualties on all sides, including between 85 000 and 91 000 fatalities, but exclude those who died from gas-related injuries years after the end of the war (*16*). The use of poison gas, including mustard gas, during warfare was prohibited by the Geneva Protocol of 1925 and the Chemical Weapons Convention of 1993, which also banned the development, production and stockpiling of such weapons.

The largest chemical weapons attack against a civilian population in modern times occurred in 1988, when Iraqi military forces repeatedly used mustard gas and other chemical agents against Kurds in northern Iraq. In the worst attack, on the Kurdish city of Halabja in March 1988, groups of aircraft flying many sorties repeatedly dropped chemical bombs. About 5000 people were killed and 65 000 others suffered severe skin and respiratory diseases and other consequences such birth defects and cancer (*17, 18*).

Biological agents

The potential of organisms used as weapons of biological warfare or bioterrorism was graphically illustrated, albeit unintentionally, by an accident involving anthrax in the former Soviet Union in 1979. The accident in Sverdlovsk, 1400 km east of Moscow, remains the largest documented outbreak of human inhalation anthrax. The number of people who died as a result has been estimated at between 45 and 100, among a total of up to 358 cases. In fatal cases, the interval between onset of symptoms and death averaged three days.

Attributed at first by government officials to the consumption of contaminated meat, it was later shown to have been caused by the accidental release of anthrax spores from a Soviet military microbiology facility. Epidemiological data revealed that most victims worked or lived in a narrow zone extending from the military facility to the southern city limit. Further south, livestock died of anthrax along the zone's extended axis. The zone paralleled the northerly wind that prevailed shortly before the outbreak. Antibiotics and vaccines were used to treat those affected and to bring the outbreak under control (*19, 20*).

Table 2.1 Examples of major chemical incidents (1974–2006)

Year	Location	Type of incident	Chemical(s) involved	Deaths	Injured	Evacuated
1974	Flixborough, United Kingdom	Chemical plant (explosion)	Cyclohexane	28	104	3000
1976	Seveso, Italy	Chemical plant (explosion)	Dioxin		193	226 000
1979	Novosibirsk, Russian Federation	Chemical plant (explosion)	Uncharacterized	300		
1981	Madrid, Spain	Foodstuff contamination (oil)	Uncharacterized	430	20 000	220 000
1982	Tacoa, Venezuela (Bolivarian Republic of)	Tank (explosion)	Fuel oil	153	20 000	40 000
1984	San Juanico, Mexico	Tank (explosion)	Liquified petroleum gas (LPG)	452	4248	200 000
1984	Bhopal, India	Chemical plant (leak)	Methyl isocyanate	2800	50 000	200 000
1992	Kwangju, Democratic People's Republic of Korea	Gas store (explosion)	LPG		163	20 000
1993	Bangkok, Thailand	Toy factory (fire)	Plastics	240	547	
1993	Remeios, Colombia	Spillage	Crude oil	430		
1996	Haiti	Poisoned medicine	Diethylene glycol	>60		
1998	Yaoundé, Cameroon	Transport accident	Petroleum products	220	130	
2000	Kinshasa, Democratic Republic of the Congo	Munitions depot (explosion)	Munitions	109	216	
2000	Enschede, Netherlands	Factory (explosion)	Fireworks	20	950	
2001	Toulouse, France	Factory (explosion)	Ammonium nitrate	30	>2500	
2002	Lagos, Nigeria	Munitions depot (explosion)	Munitions	1000		
2003	Gaoqiao, China	Gas well (release)	Hydrogen sulphide	240	9000	64 000
2005	Huaian, China	Truck (release)	Chlorine	27	300	10 000
2005	Graniteville, United States of America	Train tanker (release)	Chlorine	9	250	5400
2006	Abidjan, Côte d'Ivoire	Toxic waste	Hydrogen sulphide, mercaptans, sodium hydroxide	10	>100 000[a]	

[a] The number of consultations, not necessarily the number of people made directly ill.

Data source: (22). Data from 2000 onwards from the Major Hazard Incident Data Service (MHIDAS), Health and Safety Executive, London, United Kingdom, except for Goaqiao and Abidjan, which are from WHO.

it is from some of the larger scale incidents that the world has learned better how to prevent and respond to chemical and radioactive threats through industrial advances and diplomatic relations (see Table 2.1). Two major industrial accidents, a natural phenomenon and a forest fire are described below, all of which point to the necessity for a global response network for effective surveillance and early warning so as to mitigate the adverse effects of such occurrences.

Industrial accidents

One of the world's worst chemical accidents occurred around midnight on 2 December 1984, in the city of Bhopal in central India. A deadly cloud containing the toxic gas methyl isocyanate spilled from Union Carbide's large pesticide plant while most of the population of nearly 900 000 people were asleep (*23*).

The exact figures for the number of people killed and injured by the gas are disputed. According to official Indian figures, nearly 3000 people died in the first few hours of the accident, while hundreds of thousands were harmed, and more than 15 000 people have since died from cancer and other diseases (*23, 24*). Some estimates, however, have put the numbers much higher, suggesting that 10 000 people died initially and over 20 000 subsequently (*25*). Officially, it is estimated that about 120 000 people continue to suffer from chronic respiratory, ophthalmic, reproductive, endocrine, gastrointestinal, musculoskeletal, neurological and psychological disorders associated with the event. The release of gas also caused hundreds of thousands of people to flee the city and the polluted local environment.

The emergency and local health services were overwhelmed by the event at Bhopal. Lack of information about the identity of the gas, its health effects and the necessary clinical management and mitigation measures contributed to enormous health consequences. The acute industrial accident triggered a long-term crisis for the entire population of Bhopal, the Government of India and the industries involved. The health, economic and environmental consequences of the catastrophe are still being felt today.

Could a similar incident happen again? The answer is almost certainly yes. Chemical production and use has increased nearly tenfold worldwide over the last 30 years, and this is particularly true in developing countries (*26*). Several governments have learned from events such as Bhopal – and the accident at Seveso, Italy, where large amounts of dioxins were released into the environment in 1976 – and have introduced regulations to prevent and prepare for major chemical accidents. Poorer nations, however, are still struggling with a lack of technical capacity and regulatory infrastructure to ensure safe chemical management. In some countries with good technical capacity, the rapid pace of industrialization is outstripping the implementation of effective control measures. Increasing urbanization in such countries is exposing growing numbers of people to the risk of chemical incidents as they settle in close proximity to hazardous installations. This particularly affects the poorer segments of society who have little choice about where to live.

On 26 April 1986, explosions at reactor No. 4 of the nuclear power plant at Chernobyl in Ukraine, a republic of the former Soviet Union at that time, led to the release of huge amounts of radioactive materials into the atmosphere. These materials were deposited mainly over countries in Europe, but especially over large areas of Belarus, the Russian Federation and Ukraine. An estimated 350 000 clean-up workers or "liquidators" from the army, power plant staff, local police and fire services were initially involved in containing and cleaning up the radioactive debris during 1986–1987. About 240 000 liquidators received the highest radiation doses while conducting major mitigation activities within the 30 km zone around the reactor.

Later, the number of registered liquidators rose to 600 000, though only a small fraction of these were exposed to high levels of radiation. In the first half of 1986, 116 000 people were evacuated from the area surrounding the Chernobyl reactor to non-contaminated areas. Another 230 000 people were relocated in subsequent years. At the present time, about 5 million people live in areas of Belarus, the Russian Federation and Ukraine with levels of radioactive caesium deposition more than 37 kBq/m^2 (*27*). Among them, about 270 000 inhabitants continue to live in areas classified by their governments as strictly controlled zones, where radioactive caesium contamination exceeds 555 kBq/m^2.

In 2006, as the world marked the 20th anniversary of the Chernobyl accident, WHO released a report assessing the health impact of the worst civil nuclear accident in history (*27*). The report provided clear recommendations for future research directions and public health measures for national authorities of Belarus, the Russian Federation and Ukraine, the countries most affected by fall-out from the reactor explosion. More than 4000 thyroid cancer cases have been reported in these countries in children and adolescents for the period 1990–2002. This is significantly more than would be expected, yet precise estimates of risk are still unclear. Approximately 40% of these cases were detected through screening programmes and may otherwise have gone undetected (*27*). New thyroid cancer cases are likely to be reported in the coming decades.

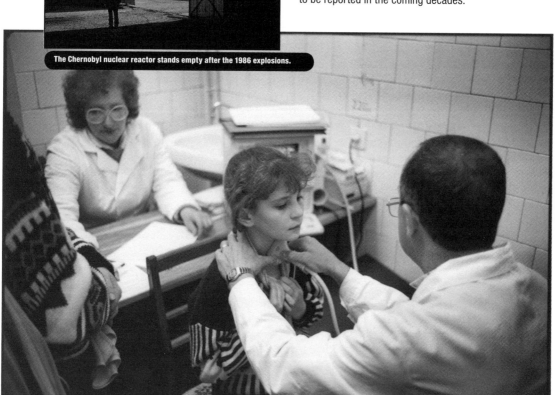

The Chernobyl nuclear reactor stands empty after the 1986 explosions.

A child of Chernobyl is examined by medical staff after the accident.

The same report revealed that the most serious long-term public health impact is in the area of mental health (*27*). In addition to the lack of reliable information provided to people affected in the first few years after the accident, there was widespread mistrust of official information and the false attribution of most health problems to radiation exposure from Chernobyl. The necessary evacuation and relocation proved a deeply traumatic experience for many people: their social networks were disrupted and they had no possibility of returning to their homes. In addition, many had to face the social stigma associated with being an "exposed person"; this stigma continues and has led to increases in risk-taking behaviour, depression and other neurological and psychological disorders.

WHO recommends that both key professionals and the general public should be provided with accurate information about the health consequences of the Chernobyl disaster, as part of efforts to revitalize the affected areas. WHO continues its efforts to support improvements in health care for affected populations through the establishment of telemedicine and educational programmes, and by supporting research.

Natural phenomena

Chemical poisoning of large numbers of people caused by a natural event rather than an industrial accident occurred in August 1986, when about 1.6 million tons of CO_2 gas were suddenly expelled from Lake Nyos, in the North-West Province of Cameroon. This event was the result of a natural phenomenon that occurred when CO_2 gas on the bed of the lake was suddenly forced into the atmosphere as a result of a large landslide into the lake. Because CO_2 is heavier than air, the gaseous mass hugged the ground surface and descended valleys along the north side of the crater at about 50 km per hour. The thick cloud covered a distance of 20 km, suffocating up to 1800 people living in the villages of Nyos, Kam, Cha and Subum (*28*, *29*). Animals were also killed, including 3500 livestock.

Although a high number of casualties might seem unavoidable following such a sudden incident, measures can be put in place for prevention and preparedness to reduce risk and population vulnerability in the future. This can be done by learning lessons from natural disasters and providing sufficient resources and technical knowledge. Unfortunately, however, this is often not the case. Rare natural events are eventually forgotten or ignored and communities can face a recurrence without being prepared.

In the case of Lake Nyos and nearby Lake Monoun, which suffered a similar eruption in 1984, pipes have been installed to allow some of the CO_2 to be siphoned off. The danger of another expulsion of CO_2 remains, however, because there are still insufficient pipes to remove the gas completely. Moreover, communities have re-settled around the lakes. Understanding the potential triggers for a catastrophic expulsion of gas, recognizing the early warning signs, and having in place an alert system could all contribute to local populations being able to avoid a recurrence of the disaster.

Forest fires produce large amounts of biomass smoke containing a mixture of particulate matter and toxic and irritant gases such as carbon monoxide, formaldehyde, acrolein, benzene, nitrogen dioxide and ozone. Wood-smoke particulates can easily be transported over great distances (30). Such small particles bypass the normal body defence mechanisms and penetrate deep into the alveoli of the lungs, harming the respiratory system.

Transboundary air pollution with smoke took place in 1997–1998, when Indonesia suffered prolonged and uncontrolled forest fires causing a dense haze that spread as far as the Philippines, Singapore and parts of Malaysia, Thailand and Viet Nam, encompassing a population of over 200 million people. About 1 million hectares of forest, plantation and scrub land, chiefly in Sumatra and Kalimantan, burned continuously from July to October 1997. This devastating event was followed by further fires in early 1998.

There have been other large-scale forest fires in Indonesia both before and since, many of which have been shown to be caused by plantation companies clearing land for agricultural use by burning vegetation (*31*). In 1997, as in some other years, the spread of the fires had been facilitated by unusually dry conditions caused by El Niño Southern Oscillation. Moreover, logging activities had also made forests more vulnerable to fire – flammable debris is left behind and the opening up of the forest canopy allows more sunlight through to dry out the forest floor.

The resulting smoke haze adversely affected the health of populations in Indonesia and neighbouring countries, causing an increase in the incidence of bronchial asthma, acute respiratory infection and conjunctivitis. In Indonesia, among the 12 360 000 people exposed to the haze, it was estimated that there were over 1 800 000 cases of bronchial asthma, bronchitis and acute respiratory infection (*32*). Health surveillance in Singapore from August to November 1997 showed a 30% increase in hospital outpatient attendance for haze-related conditions, as well as an increase in accident and emergency attendances (*33*). A study in Malaysia found significant increases in respiratory hospitalizations related to the haze, specifically those for chronic obstructive pulmonary disease and asthma. The most vulnerable group was people over the age of 65 (*34*). The long-term effects on health from exposure to the haze are yet to be determined.

Causes of acute threats to public health security include those outlined for infectious diseases, acute events that occur after war or natural disasters, and chemical or nuclear events. This chapter has provided examples of many of these causes and the consequences as seen during the last century.

Chapter 3 describes more recent events in the 21st century and increases our understanding of why border controls and international agreements are not enough – there must be strong national surveillance and response mechanisms to detect and respond to threats where and when they occur, together with global mechanisms to detect and respond should they become threats to global public health security.

REFERENCES

1. *International Health Regulations (2005)*. Article 1 Definitions. Geneva, World Health Organization, 2006.
2. Centers for Disease Control and Prevention. Pneumocystis pneumonia – Los Angeles. *Morbidity and Mortality Weekly Report*, 1982, 30:250–252.
3. *Measure DHS: overview*. Calverton, MD, Macro International Inc., Demographic and Health Surveys (http://www.measuredhs.com/topics/hiv/start.cfm, accessed 25 April 2007).
4. *Marburg haemorrhagic fever in Angola – update 7*. Geneva, World Health Organization, 2005 (http://www.who.int/csr/don/2005_04_06/en, accessed 12 April 2007).
5. *Field news – Marburg fever: epidemic still not under control*. New York, NY, Doctors without Borders, 2005 (http://www.doctorswithoutborders.org/news/2005/05-02-2005.cfm, accessed 12 April 2007).
6. *Marburg haemorrhagic fever in Angola – update 26: MOH declares outbreak over*. Geneva, World Health Organization, 2005 (http://www.who.int/csr/don/2005_11_07a/en/index.html, accessed 12 April 2007).
7. Bausch DG, Borchert M, Grein T, Roth C, Swanepoel R, Libande ML et al. Risk factors for Marburg hemorrhagic fever in Durba and Watsa, Democratic Republic of the Congo. *Emerging Infectious Diseases*, 2003, 9:1531–1537.
8. Goma Epidemiologic Group. Public health impact of Rwandan refugee crisis: what happened in Goma, Zaire, in July 1994? *Lancet*, 1995, 345:339–344.
9. Heymann DL. Emerging infections. In: Schaechter M, ed. *The desk encyclopedia of microbiology*. Amsterdam, Elsevier Academic Press, 2004.

10. Levy SB. Antibiotic resistance: an ecological imbalance. In: Chadwick DJ, Goode J, eds. *Antibiotic resistance: origins, evolution, selection and spread.* Chichester, John Wiley and Sons, 1997: (Ciba Foundation Symposium 207).

11. Fleming A. Penicillin: Nobel Lecture, 11 December 1945 (http://nobelprize.org/nobel_prizes/ medicine/laureates/1945/fleming-lecture.pdf, accessed 11 May 2007).

12. Levy SB. Antimicrobial resistance: bacteria on the defence [editorial]. *British Medical Journal*, 1998, 317:612–613.

13. *Fourth vCJD case linked with blood transfusion in UK.* Minneapolis, MN, Center for Infectious Disease Research and Policy, 2007 (http://www.cidrap.umn.edu/cidrap/content/other/bse/ news/jan2207vcjd.html, accessed 24 April 2007).

14. *FAO/WHO Global Forum on Food Safety Regulators, Marrakech, Morocco, 28-30 January 2002: Japanese encephalitis/Nipah outbreak in Malaysia.* Rome, Food and Agriculture Organization, 2002 (GF/CRD Malaysia-1; http://www.fao.org/DOCREP/MEETING/004/AB455E.HTM, accessed 18 May 2007).

15. Outbreak of Rift Valley fever, Eastern Africa, 1997-1998. *Weekly Epidemiological Record*, 1998, 73:105–109.

16. Poison gas and World War I. History Learning (http://www.historylearningsite.co.uk/poison_gas_and_world_war_one.htm, accessed 19 April 2007).

17. *Mustard gas.* New York, NY, Council on Foreign Relations, 2006 (http://www.cfr.org/ publication/9551/, accessed 19 April 2007).

18. Gosden CM. The 1988 chemical weapons attack on Halabja, Iraq. In: Yonah A, Hoenig M, eds. *Super terrorism: biological, chemical, and nuclear.* Ardsley, NY, Transnational Publishers Inc., 2001.

19. Meselson M, Guillemin J, Hugh-Jones M, Langmuir A, Popova I, Shelokov A et al. The Sverdlovsk anthrax outbreak of 1979. *Science*, 1994, 266:1202–1208.

20. Anthrax as a biological weapon, 2002: updated recommendations for management. *Journal of the American Medical Association*, 2002, 287:2236–2252.

21. International Programme on Chemical Safety (http://www.who.int/ipcs/en/, accessed on 3 April 2007).

22. *Public health and chemical incidents: guidance for national and regional policy makers in the public health/environmental health roles.* Cardiff, International Clearing House for Major Chemical Incidents, University of Wales Institute, 1999.

23. *Facts and figures.* Bhopal, Government of Madhya Pradesh, Bhopal Gas Tragedy Relief and Rehabilitation Department (http://www.mp.nic.in/bgtrrdmp/facts.htm, accessed 24 April 2007).

24. *Health effects of the toxic gas leak from the Union Carbide Methyl Isocyanate Plant in Bhopal: technical report on population-based long-term epidemiological studies (1985–1994).* New Delhi, Indian Council of Medical Research, 2004.

25. *Clouds of injustice: Bhopal disaster 20 years on.* Oxford, Amnesty International, 2004.

26. *Environmental outlook for the chemical industry.* Paris, Organisation for Economic Co-operation and Development, 2001.

27. *Health effects of the Chernobyl accident and special health care programmes.* Geneva, World Health Organization, 2006 (Fact sheet 303).

28. Baxter PJ, Kapila M, Mfonfu D. Lake Nyos disaster, Cameroon, 1986: the medical effects of large-scale emission of carbon dioxide? *British Medical Journal,* 1989, 298:1437–1441.

29. Camp V. *Lake Nyos 1986.* San Diego, State University Department of Geological Sciences, (http://www.geology.sdsu.edu/how_volcanoes_work/Nyos.html, accessed 11 March 2007).

30. Brauer M. Health impacts of biomass air pollution. In: Goh K-T et al, eds. *Health guidelines for vegetation fire events.* Geneva, World Health Organization, 1999.

31. Byron N, Shepherd G. Indonesia and the 1997-98 El Niño: fire problems and long-term solutions. *Natural Resource Perspectives*, 1998, No. 28 (http://www.odi.org.uk/NRP/28. html, accessed 11 March 2007).

32. Dawud Y. Smoke episodes and assessment of health impacts related to haze from forest fires: Indonesian experience. In: Goh K-T et al, eds. *Health guidelines for vegetation fire events.* Geneva, World Health Organization, 1999.

33. Emmanuel SC. Impact to lung health of haze from forest fires: the Singapore experience. *Respirology*, 2000, 5:175-82.

34. Mott JA et al. Cardio-respiratory hospitalizations associated with smoke exposure during the 1997 Southeast Asian forest fires. *International Journal of Hygiene and Environmental Health,* 2005, 208:75-85.

NEW
HEALTH THREATS
in the 21st century

chapter

3

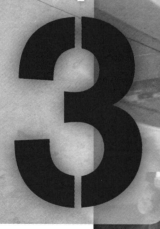

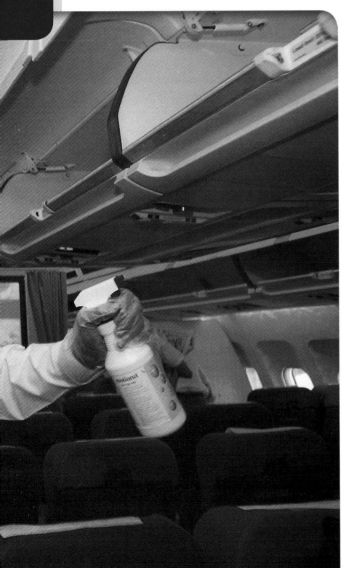

The previous chapter identified the main causes of infectious diseases and other acute events that threaten collective public health. Chapter 3 continues with a number of major events that have occurred in the first few years of the 21st century and which represent new threats to national and global public health security. The examples discussed are bioterrorism in the form of the anthrax letters in the United States in 2001, the emergence of Severe Acute Respiratory Syndrome (SARS) in 2003, and large-scale dumping of toxic chemical waste in Côte d'Ivoire in 2006.

These events demonstrate how much the world is changing in terms of its vulnerability to new threats to health. Chronologically, the first of these is the arrival of bioterrorism on the international stage with the anthrax letters attack in the United States in 2001. This was followed in 2003 by the emergence and rapid international spread of the deadly new disease SARS. The international impact of this disease contributed to the growing political will to complete the revision and strengthening of the International Health Regulations (1969), and to enable a much more proactive approach to preparedness for an expected human influenza pandemic (see Chapter 4).

In 2006, the illegal dumping of hundreds of tons of chemical waste in Côte d'Ivoire provoked tens of thousands of cases of respiratory and other illnesses, and illustrated a growing phenomenon – how globalization has exacerbated the dangers inherent in the movement and disposal of hazardous wastes. The episode, described later in this chapter, is linked to the extended response system to chemical incidents that covers such environmental health emergencies (see Chapter 2).

THE ANTHRAX LETTERS

Coming only days after the terrorist events of 11 September 2001 in the United States, the deliberate dissemination of potentially lethal anthrax spores in letters sent through the United States Postal Service (1) added the deliberate release of biological or chemical agents to the realities of life in the 21st century. Anthrax spores were found in four envelopes. In addition to the human toll – five people died among 22 cases (2) – the anthrax attack caused massive disruption of postal services in many countries around the world and had huge economic, public health and security consequences. It prompted renewed international concerns about bioterrorism, provoking countermeasures in many countries and requests for a greater advisory role by WHO that led to the updated publication of *Public health response to biological and chemical weapons: WHO guidance* (3).

36

world health report 2007
global public health security
in the 21st century

For years, the United States and other industrialized countries had lived with the fear – frequently fed by hoax calls and alarms – of just such an attack. Although there was no evidence that they had been used, it was well known that stocks of biological weapons, including anthrax, were held by a number of countries. Investigations into the accidental release of anthrax from a military biological weapons facility in the former Soviet Union in 1979 showed how lethal it could be (see Chapter 2).

In 1990, during the Gulf War, the United States Government's concern about potential anthrax attacks led to the vaccination of more than 100 000 military personnel. In 1995, this concern was again aroused when the United Nations Special Commission indicated that Iraq had been developing and testing anthrax weapons during the Kuwait War. In 1998, a programme was initiated to vaccinate all United States military personnel, and government agencies were given directives for responding to possible deliberate biological or chemical attacks on civilian centres.

Starting in 1997, the United States experienced an increasing number of anthrax threats and hoaxes that, by the end of 1998, were regular occurrences. Prominent among these were envelopes containing various powders and materials, which were sent through the mail to abortion and reproductive health clinics, government offices and other locations. Until the events of 11 September 2001, none of these materials had tested positive for pathogenic *Bacillus anthracis* and there had not been a case of inhalational anthrax in the United States since 1976.

By 2001, with federal assistance, most American state governments and authorities of large cities had begun to develop plans to deal with bioterrorism and many had staged mock attacks to test local emergency response capacity. Effective medical measures for prevention and treatment of the two forms of the disease – cutaneous and inhalational anthrax – were established and published in the medical literature well before the anthrax letter attacks.

Nevertheless the anthrax letters – dated 11 September 2001 and postmarked seven days later – caused huge public alarm and prompted a massive public health response. In the end, a total of 22 persons are thought to have been infected: 11 each with cutaneous and inhalation anthrax. The five patients who died were all infected with inhalation anthrax (*3*). Twenty of the 22 patients were exposed to work sites that were found to be contaminated with anthrax spores; nine had worked in mail processing facilities through which the anthrax letters had passed. Drugs were made available on an emergency basis to some 32 000 people who were potentially exposed. Altogether, about 3.75 million antimicrobial tablets were distributed. People presumed to be at higher risk were advised to remain on a prolonged course of 60 days and were also given the option of anthrax vaccination. The CDC sent emergency teams of epidemiologists and laboratory and logistics staff to support local, state and federal health investigations and medicine distribution.

The collection and testing of environmental and clinical samples, as well as materials from suspicious incidents and hoaxes, placed an immense burden on the CDC, public health laboratories throughout the country and government agencies. The magnitude of the clinical and environmental testing undertaken would have quickly overwhelmed the nation's capacity had a significant investment not already been made in expanding laboratory training and capacity through a system called the Laboratory Response Network (LRN). The network links state and local public health laboratories with advanced capacity laboratories, including clinical, military, veterinary and agricultural laboratories, and those for testing water and food.

One legacy of the crisis was the introduction of permanent decontamination, detection and security equipment at mail processing facilities across the country. In order to reduce potentially contaminated dust and aerosols from the atmosphere in its centres, the Postal Service introduced some 16 000 high efficiency particulate air filter vacuum machines and, as a precaution, routinely sterilizes mail going to federal agencies by electron-beam irradiation. For the two fiscal years 2003 and 2004, US$ 1.7 billion was budgeted for additional modifications and improvements in the government's ability to protect the health of postal workers and to prevent pathogens and other hazardous substances from being distributed through the mail.

Even though the deliberate release of the anthrax was directed at one country, it had region-wide effect in the Americas. This was especially so as public health infrastructures had to divert resources to face an overwhelming demand for laboratory tests for suspected tainted postal items, personal protective equipment and for the decontamination of facilities.

Occurring as it did so soon after the September 2001 terrorist attacks, the anthrax offensive prompted a profound rethinking of threats to national and international security. It showed the potential of bioterrorism to cause not just death and disability, but social and economic disruption on an enormous scale both in the United States and internationally.

A simultaneous concern was that smallpox – a debilitating, disfiguring and frequently deadly disease that was eradicated in 1979[1] – could be used over 20 years later as one of the most effective biological weapons conceivable. This was of particular concern given that mass smallpox vaccination had been discontinued after eradication, thus leaving unimmunized populations susceptible. An expert who had led the smallpox eradication campaign warned in June 1999, "If used as a biological weapon, smallpox represents a serious threat to civilian populations because of its case fatality rate of 30% or more among unvaccinated persons and the absence of specific therapy. Although smallpox has long been feared as the most devastating of all infectious diseases, its potential for devastation today is far greater than at any previous time" (4).

WHO has participated in international discussions and bioterrorism desktop exercises, arguing that the surest way to detect a deliberately caused outbreak is to strengthen the systems used for detecting natural outbreaks, as the epidemiological and laboratory principles are fundamentally the same. Consideration of the appropriate response to a biological attack, especially to the smallpox virus, served to test – on a global scale – the GOARN mechanisms recently introduced by WHO. In addition, the debate in medical journals, the media, and security and defence circles helped to persuade political leaders that improved national capacities for disease surveillance and response are directly relevant to national and international security.

SARS: VULNERABILITY REVEALED

In 2003, SARS – the first severe new disease of the 21st century – confirmed fears, generated by the bioterrorism threat, that a new or unfamiliar pathogen would have profound national and international implications for public health and economic security. SARS defines the features that give a disease international significance as a public health security threat: it spreads from person to person, requires no vector, displays

---

[1] The global eradication of smallpox was certified by a commission of eminent scientists in December 1979 based on intensive in-country verification activities. It was subsequently endorsed by the World Health Assembly in 1980.

no particular geographical affinity, incubates silently for more than a week, mimics the symptoms of many other diseases, takes its heaviest toll on hospital staff, and kills around 10% of those infected. These features enable it to spread easily along the routes of international air travel, placing every city with an international airport at risk of imported cases (see Figure 3.1).

New, deadly and initially poorly understood, SARS incited a degree of public anxiety that brought travel to affected areas to a virtual standstill and drained billions of dollars from economies across entire regions. Box 3.1 details the economic costs of the SARS epidemic and projects the possible economic consequences of a large influenza pandemic.

SARS demonstrated that the risks and dangers to health arising from new diseases have indeed been increased by the ways in which nations and their populations interact globally. It showed the magnitude of damage that an emerging disease with the appropriate features can cause in a world where airlines carried an estimated 2.1 billion passengers in 2006 (7), where financial markets and businesses are tightly intertwined, and where information is instantly accessible (see Figure 3.2).

The emergency response and the level of media attention stimulated by SARS were on a scale that challenged public and political perceptions of the risks associated with emerging and epidemic-prone diseases (see Box 3.2). The outbreak raised the profile of public health to new heights. Neither the public nor government officials at the highest levels could ignore the adverse effects that a health problem was having on economies, societies, politics and the international image of countries. Not every

Figure 3.1   Probable SARS transmission on flight CA112 in March 2003

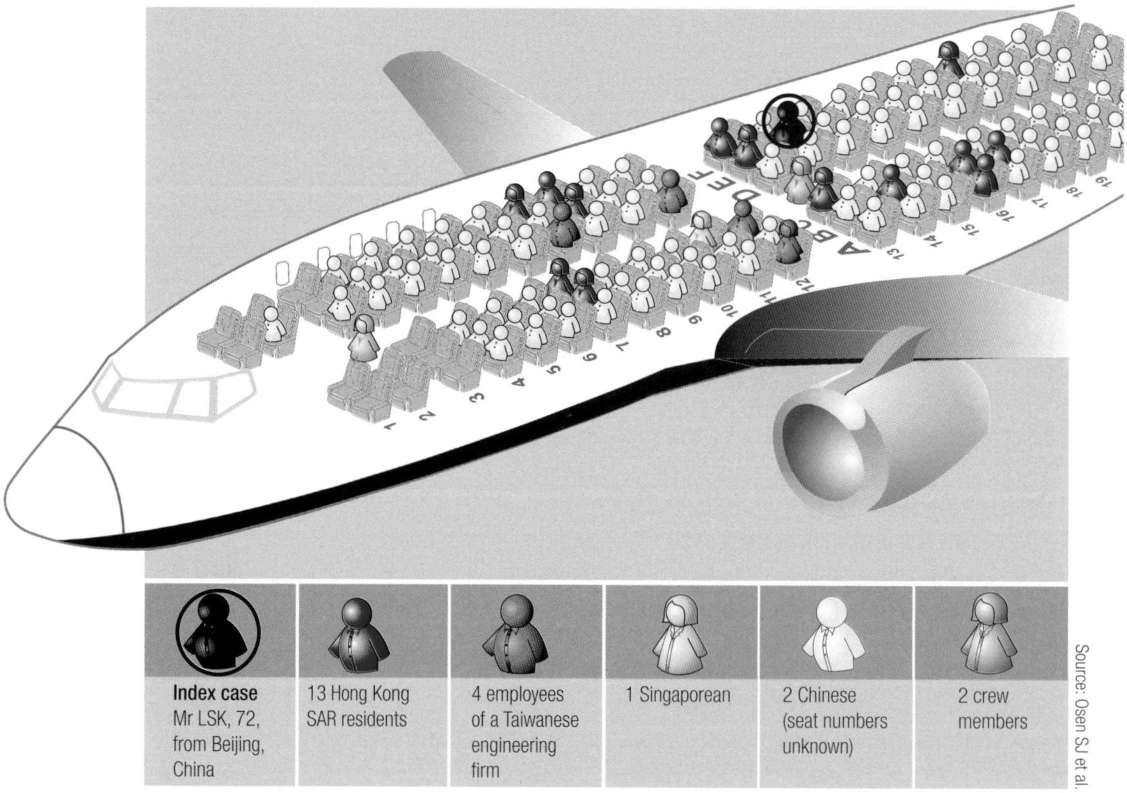

| Index case Mr LSK, 72, from Beijing, China | 13 Hong Kong SAR residents | 4 employees of a Taiwanese engineering firm | 1 Singaporean | 2 Chinese (seat numbers unknown) | 2 crew members |

Source: Osen SJ et al.

A total of 22 passengers, and the index case, met WHO's definition of a probable case of SARS.

Box 3.1 Economic impact of SARS and influenza pandemics

The 2003 epidemic of SARS could possibly have been a global pandemic responsible for millions of deaths. Instead, using classic surveillance and epidemiological response techniques, the epidemic was limited to 8422 cases with a case-fatality rate of 11% (*5*). Even so, the estimated cost of the epidemic to Asian countries was US$ 20 billion in gross domestic product (GDP) terms for 2003, or a more dramatic US$ 60 billion of gross expenditure and business losses (*6*).

The main drivers of the economic impact of SARS were tourism and consumer confidence for non-essential spending. The actual number of SARS cases was relatively small,

seen in the case of SARS, as illustrated below.

If a pandemic were to persist for over a year, as has been predicted, the long-term consequences in terms of job loss and bankruptcy would continue to produce hardship for many years. The longer the pandemic remained active, the greater the damage in terms of losses in productivity, along with hospitalization and other health-care expenditures.

Of course, the larger the pandemic, in terms of proportion of the population infected, the greater the economic impact. For infection rates up to 1% of the world's population, a decrease in global GDP of 5% could be expected,

Estimated economic impact of pandemic influenza

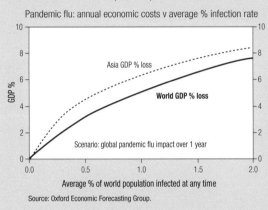

Pandemic flu: annual economic costs v average % infection rate

Asia GDP % loss

World GDP % loss

Scenario: global pandemic flu impact over 1 year

Average % of world population infected at any time

Source: Oxford Economic Forecasting Group.

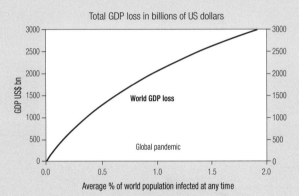

Total GDP loss in billions of US dollars

World GDP loss

Global pandemic

Average % of world population infected at any time

but the fear of transmission caused foreign tourists to choose alternative holiday locations, and the local population felt safer avoiding restaurants and other public leisure venues. These sectors of the economy are significant contributors to the GDP of many countries.

Both human and economic consequences were mostly confined to the second quarter of 2003. Although the duration and economic impact of the outbreak were checked by strong leadership and coordinated international public health action, this success invites the question "what could have happened?"

The total cost of SARS to Asian countries breaks down to over US$ 2 million per person infected. A true influenza pandemic would certainly last longer than three months, but the economic implications of an influenza outbreak lasting a year or more are not a simple multiplication of what was

with an additional loss of 1% per additional percentage increase in infection rate (*6*). Once a critical infection rate was reached, the cumulative economic disruption would produce a shut-down of the global economy, similar to that seen in the United Kingdom's agricultural economy following the 2001 outbreak of foot and mouth disease but, in this case, on a global scale (*6*).

The potential calamity caused by a global influenza pandemic justifies naming the control of such a pandemic a global public good. Current stocks of vaccines and anti-viral medications are not adequate in any country, let alone in developing countries. Pandemics, by definition, have no respect for national and regional borders. The health impact of the pandemic influenza virus will be shared, as will the economic losses.

country felt threatened by the prospect of deliberate biological attack, but every country was concerned by the arrival of a disease like SARS.

SARS also highlighted the fact that the danger arising from emerging diseases is universal. No country is automatically protected – by virtue of its wealth or its high levels of education, standards of living and health care, or equipment and personnel at border crossings – from either the arrival of a new disease on its territory or the subsequent disruption this can cause. SARS was, to a large extent, a disease of prosperous urban centres. Contrary to expectations, it spread most efficiently in sophisticated city hospitals.

SARS did not become endemic in humans or gradually fade away. Its spread was halted less than four months after it was first recognized as an international threat – an unprecedented achievement for public health on a global scale. Had SARS been allowed to establish a foothold in a resource-poor setting, it is doubtful whether the demanding measures, facilities and technologies needed to interrupt chains of transmission could have been fully deployed. If SARS had become permanently established as yet another indigenous epidemic threat, it is not difficult to imagine the consequences for global public health security in a world still struggling to cope with HIV/AIDS.

DUMPING OF TOXIC CHEMICALS

As well as the international mobility of people, the global movement of products can have serious health consequences. The potentially deadly risks of the international movement and disposal of hazardous wastes as an element of global trade were vividly illustrated in Côte d'Ivoire in August 2006. Over 500 tons of chemical waste were unloaded from a cargo ship and illegally dumped by trucks at different sites in

Figure 3.2 Direct economic impact of selected infectious disease outbreaks, 1990–2003[a]

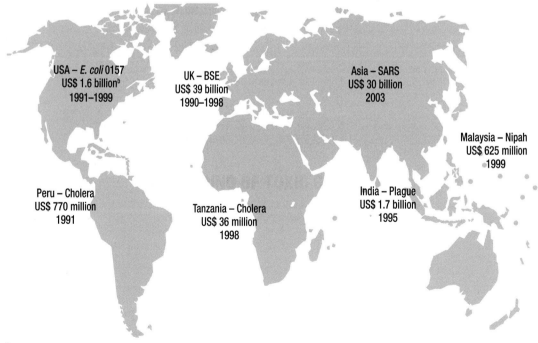

USA – *E. coli* 0157
US$ 1.6 billion[b]
1991–1999

UK – BSE
US$ 39 billion
1990–1998

Asia – SARS
US$ 30 billion
2003

Malaysia – Nipah
US$ 625 million
1999

Peru – Cholera
US$ 770 million
1991

Tanzania – Cholera
US$ 36 million
1998

India – Plague
US$ 1.7 billion
1995

[a] Excludes economic impact of human sickness and death.
[b] Date source: (8).

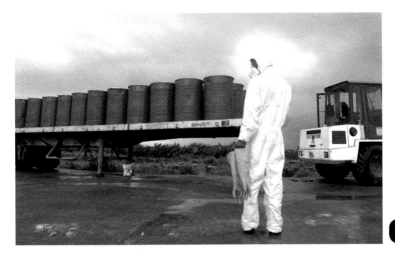

Toxicological dumping in Côte d'Ivoire –
the clean up begins.

Box 3.2 The role of the mass media in risk perceptions

News travels fast – and it has never travelled faster than in today's world of instant information. The mass media have a powerful influence on people's perceptions of risks, whether from a new disease epidemic, deliberate attacks or natural catastrophes. The Internet, television, radio, newspapers and magazines are the most influential sources of everyday information on risks to health.

How should the media evaluate and communicate information on health risks such as avian influenza or SARS? Such situations challenge the media to be responsible when dealing with complicated scientific issues and conflicting political goals. What information should be conveyed? How fully should uncertainties and controversies be explained to the public?

In covering health issues, the media perform two major functions: they explain and report scientific information and government policies for the public and, at the same time, reflect the concerns of the general public. Health-related events such as chemical accidents, medical research discoveries, communicable disease epidemics and safety defects in new medicines are all likely to make headlines. Government press releases, scientists and international scientific journals are often their main sources of information. Journalists tend to use the best-organized sources and those press releases that encapsulate technical information in lay terms. In addition, international news organizations frequently syndicate health-risk stories around the world (9).

According to a study by the Nuffield Trust, mass communication can either heighten levels of anxiety or provide reassurance at times of acute public health events. Authorities such as governments may use the mass media, but can seldom keep control of the information delivered. They have to strike a difficult balance between saying too much and saying too little: one course of action may cause an overreaction, the other may seem complacent (10).

Mass communication has both a positive and negative potential for risk perception. When no information about health risks is provided through official channels, the media will find it elsewhere and their reports may create or heighten a sense of anxiety. For those in authority, doing or saying nothing has become a dangerous strategy. For example, early reports of a disease outbreak are often alarmist, as was shown in the case of the SARS outbreak in 2003. This can establish a baseline of accepted "facts" or beliefs that may be difficult to correct when more – and especially more accurate – information becomes available.

"On the other hand, mass communications can be used to reassure the public. In this respect, the role of WHO during SARS is instructive," says the Nuffield Trust study. "As a trusted international body it was able to use mass communication to inform and reassure anxious publics. Indeed, the speed of modern communication can even be a reassurance in itself: as SARS demonstrated, modern communication technology allowed the rapid exchange of information which allowed better preventative action, while the exchange of scientific data through secure web sites, etc. allowed the SARS genome to be identified remarkably quickly."

The study says health professionals – and in particular professional bodies – have a role to play in reassuring the public over the risks involved, but such responses need to be agile and perceived as independent and authoritative.

and around Abidjan. One month after the dumping, almost 85 000 consultations had been recorded at different medical facilities in relation to the chemical incident and its consequences: 69 people had been admitted to hospital and eight deaths had been attributed to the event.

The composition of the "slop" unloaded from the vessel was initially unknown, but it caused eye, nose and throat irritation, breathing difficulties, headaches, nausea and vomiting, and growing anxiety among thousands of people. The most severe cases presented with respiratory distress, dehydration, and nose and intestinal bleeding. In addition to the eight deaths attributed to the incident initially, more are suspected to have occurred due to the worsening of pre-existing medical conditions such as asthma, respiratory conditions or cardiovascular disease. Even several weeks after the dumping, the foul odours persisted at certain times of the day, and people with nose, throat and skin irritation, as well as malaise, nausea and gastrointestinal effects, were still seeking medical attention at the hospitals, where free care and medication was provided.

The waste was eventually identified as a mixture of sodium hydroxide, phenols, mercaptanes, hydrogen sulphide, hydrocarbons and other chemicals used to clean oil transporters' tanks, all of which can have severe toxic and caustic effects requiring symptomatic treatment.

This incident had important public health, social and economic consequences. It occurred in a climate of social unrest and political instability that was further intensified by the reactions of the people. Street demonstrations and violent incidents occurred every day.

Thousands of people arrived at the medical centres with either health complaints or – especially in the case of pregnant women – fears about the future consequences of exposure to the chemicals, stretching the provision of normal medical care to the limit. Pharmaceutical stocks, X-ray plates, laboratory reagents and other supplies were soon scarce. As the medical personnel were overwhelemed, more staff had to be recruited in order to deal with the overflow of consultations. The public health system was in crisis and unable to provide the medical care required by the population.

In addition, there was increasing local and international concern about potential water and food contamination, as dead fish were reported in the lagoon and vegetables grown near contaminated sites were being sold in the local markets. Some of the contaminated areas that happened to be waste disposal sites were closed for security reasons and, as a consequence, the normal garbage collection system was disrupted and domestic rubbish began piling up in different areas of the city.

The situation required government intervention at the highest level as well as the support of national and international organizations. WHO provided technical advice to country authorities, acquired pharmaceuticals and other resources for the over-worked hospitals, supplied computers and case data forms, prepared and circulated information notes, and established contacts with other organizations of the United Nations system.

Neighbouring countries were concerned that rivers and the sea would carry contamination and they remained on the alert. One of the main international concerns was that the ship transporting the waste had sailed from northern Europe and had called at a number of ports, including some others in western Africa, on its way to Côte d'Ivoire. It was unclear in the aftermath of the incident whether it had taken on, or discharged, chemical waste at any of those ports of call.

In today's world, public health security needs to be provided through coordinated action and cooperation between and within governments, the corporate sector, civil society, the media and individuals. No single institution or country has all the capabilities needed to respond to international public health emergencies caused by epidemics, natural disasters, environmental emergencies, chemical or biological attacks, or new and emerging infectious diseases. Only by detecting and reporting problems in their earliest hours can the most appropriate experts and resources be deployed to prevent or halt the international spread of disease.

Chapter 4 examines recent experience in avian influenza alert and response, the new threat of XDR-TB and natural disasters caused by extreme weather events.

REFERENCES

1. *Diffuse security threats: technologies for mail sanitization exist, but challenges remain.* Washington, DC, United States General Accounting Office, 2002 (GAO–02–365).
2. Jernigan DB, Raghunathan PL, Bell BP, Brechner R, Bresnitz EA, Butler JC et al. Investigation of bioterrorism-related anthrax, United States, 2001: epidemiologic findings. *Online Emerging Infectious Diseases*, 8 October 2002 (http://www.cdc.gov/ncidod/EID/vol8no10/02-0353. htm, accessed 25 April 2007).
3. *Public health response to biological and chemical weapons: WHO guidance.* (2nd ed. of *Health aspects of biological and chemical weapons, 1970*). Geneva, World Health Organization, 2004 (http://www.who.int/csr/delibepidemics/biochemguide/en/index.html, accessed 15 May 2007).
4. Fenner F, Henderson DA, Arita I, Ježek Z, Ladnyi ID. *Smallpox and its eradication.* Geneva, World Health Organization, 1988.
5. *Summary table of SARS cases by country, 1 November 2002–7 August 2003.* Geneva, World Health Organization (http://www.who.int/csr/sars/country/2003_08_15/en/index. html, accessed 11 December 2006).
6. Rossi V, Walker J. *Assessing the economic impact and costs of flu pandemics originating in Asia.* Oxford, Oxford Economic Forecasting, 2005.
7. *Fact sheet: IATA.* Geneva, International Air Transport Association, 2007 (http://www.iata. org/pressroom/facts_figures/fact_sheets/iata.htm, accessed 10 May 2007).
8. Marsh TL, Shroeder TC, Mintert J. Impacts of meat product recalls on consumer demand in the USA. *Applied Economics,* 2004, 36:897–909.
9. *The world health report 2002 – reducing risks, promoting healthy life.* Geneva, World Health Organization, 2002.
10. *Health, security and the risk society.* London, Nuffield Trust Global Health Progamme, 2005.

LEARNING
LESSONS
thinking ahead

chapter

4

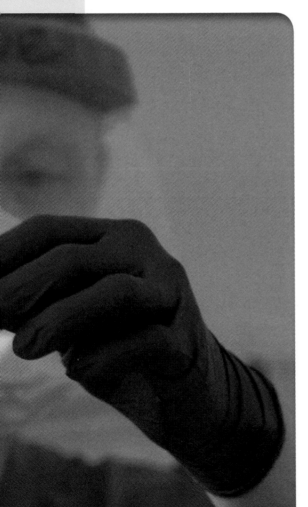

Chapter 4 is devoted to potential public health emergencies of international concern, the most feared of which remains pandemic influenza. The response to this threat has already been proactive and has been a rare opportunity to prepare for a pandemic, and possibly to prevent the threat becoming a reality.

The IHR (2005) provide the framework for this approach through national core capacity strengthening and a call for collective response to public health emergencies of international concern. Chapter 4 examines lessons being learned from experiences gained through the early application of IHR (2005) in the pandemic influenza alert, and their potential application in situations such as extensively drug-resistant tuberculosis (XDR-TB) in southern Africa and the threat of the international spread of poliomyelitis.

These latter two situations are examples of the type of public health events that would evoke use of the decision instrument of IHR (2005) to assess the need to notify WHO of a public health emergency of international concern (see Chapter 5) and, if deemed necessary, would require a collective public health response.

PANDEMIC INFLUENZA: THE MOST FEARED SECURITY THREAT

In sharp contrast to the entirely reactive response to the SARS outbreak of 2003, the response to the threat of a new influenza pandemic has already been emphatically proactive – facilitated by early implementation of IHR (2005). This has been a rare opportunity to prevent the threat becoming a reality by taking full advantage of advance warning and by testing a model for pandemic planning and preparedness.

The threat of pandemic influenza cannot be fully appreciated, however, without first understanding its relationship to seasonal influenza. Every year, human influenza rapidly spreads around the world in seasonal epidemics, typically resulting in an estimated three to five million cases of severe illness and between 250 000 and 500 000 deaths.

Most deaths currently associated with influenza in industrialized countries occur among people over 65 years of age. The causative seasonal influenza viruses are divided into two groups: A and B. Influenza A has two subtypes of seasonal viruses which are important for humans: A(H3N2) and A(H1N1), the former of which is currently associated with most deaths.

Seasonal influenza viruses frequently undergo minor genetic changes, known as "antigenic drift". These changes require annual reformulation of influenza vaccines to protect populations in different regions of the world. The most effective vaccines for seasonal influenza are those that are specifically produced for the currently circulating virus.

Seasonal influenza outbreaks typically first appear in the East and then travel westward. Viruses detected early in Asia are therefore analysed and used to predict the components used in the preparation of the vaccines for the subsequent influenza season.

For the past 50 years, genetic information on the constantly changing strains of circulating influenza viruses obtained from freely shared and exchanged viruses from countries, and on the epidemiological trends of influenza infection has been gathered by an extensive surveillance network (the

Global Influenza Surveillance Network) administered by WHO. The network currently consists of more than 118 National Influenza Centres in over 89 countries, and four WHO Collaborating Centres in Australia, Japan, the United Kingdom and the United States (see Figure 4.1). National Influenza Centres ensure that representative viral insolates are transferred to the Collaborating Centres for immediate strain identification.

WHO also administers FluNet, an Internet-based geographical information system with a remote data entry component, which allows real time access to the latest country-specific data on circulating strains and epidemiological trends. Launched in 1997, FluNet contributes to global influenza surveillance by giving researchers and others a tool to access information on influenza activity (1).

Apart from guiding the annual composition of recommended seasonal influenza vaccines, the Global Influenza Surveillance Network and FluNet operate as a global early warning system on the emergence of influenza variants and new strains. The network is reliable and sufficiently sensitive to pick up any new influenza virus with pandemic potential and any outbreak of unusually severe illness and rapid spread. It played a key role in the early detection, investigation and containment of the 1997 outbreak of H5N1 avian influenza in humans in China, Hong Kong Special Administrative Region.

Human cases and deaths related to H5N1 avian influenza were first reported in Hong Kong SAR in 1997. By 6 June 2007, the cumulative number of human cases reported to WHO had risen to 310, including 189 deaths. Although relatively few in number, they are symbolic of an emerging epidemic disease that presents a major threat to life, economies and security. While the timing and severity of a pandemic cannot be predicted, the world has been given the unprecedented advantage of advance warning that a pandemic may be near. This advantage is being fully exploited to enhance global preparedness under the framework of IHR (2005).

Although H5N1 was first isolated from humans in 1997, it was intensified surveillance for a recurrence of SARS in 2003 and 2004 that first detected a cluster of young

Figure 4.1 WHO influenza surveillance network

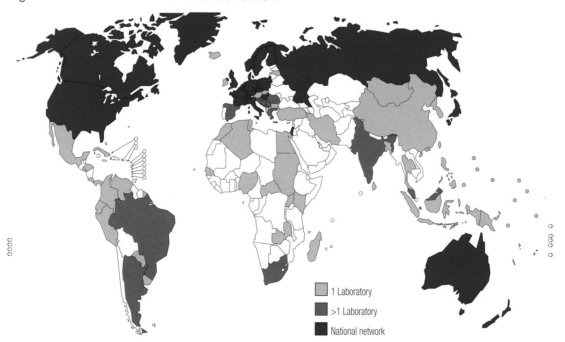

1 Laboratory

>1 Laboratory

National network

children with H5N1 infection, many of whom had died from severe respiratory disease at a paediatric hospital in Hanoi, Viet Nam. This outbreak of human cases of avian influenza was caused by the highly pathogenic H5N1 virus and accompanied by huge outbreaks in poultry. It was a signal of what might follow.

Coming on the heels of the SARS outbreak, the prospect of an influenza pandemic sparked immediate alarm around the world and with good reason. Far more contagious, spread by coughing and sneezing and transmitted during an incubation period too short to allow for contact tracing and isolation, pandemic influenza would extend the devastating consequences that had been seen with SARS in Asia and Canada to every corner of the world within a matter of months. Moreover, if a fully transmissible pandemic virus emerged, the spread of the disease could not be prevented. Even a measure as drastic as a complete ban on international travel might, at best, delay arrival of the virus in a country by a few weeks.

Based on experiences with past pandemics, illness affecting around 25% of the world's population has been predicted by some experts. This calculates to more than 1.5 billion people – more than the combined populations of China and the United States. Should this prove accurate, the impact that the first influenza pandemic since the turn of the century would have on national and international public health, and on economic and political security, can easily be foreseen. Even if the virus caused relatively mild symptoms, the economic and social disruption arising from sudden surges of illness in so many people – occurring almost simultaneously throughout the world – would be enormous.

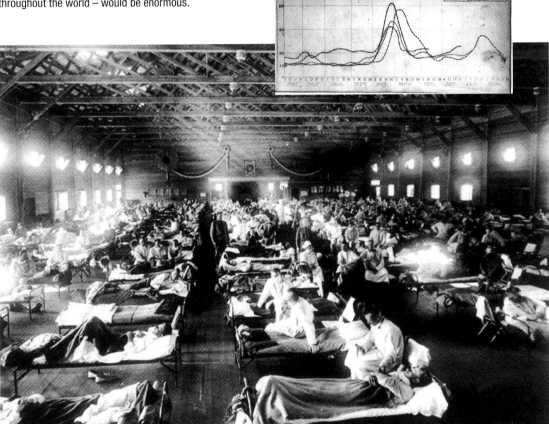

An emergency hospital in the United States during the 1918–1919 influenza pandemic.

With so much at stake, the expanding outbreaks in poultry and human cases in Viet Nam, followed within days by cases in Thailand, stimulated a flurry of research activity involving epidemiologists, clinicians, virologists and veterinarians. Researchers combed through the histories of past pandemics searching for clues that could shed light on what might lie in store and how best to prepare. Industry accelerated its efforts to develop a pandemic vaccine and to augment manufacturing capacity for the principal antiviral drug, oseltamivir. The WHO Global Influenza Surveillance Network continued to identify human infections with avian influenza viruses. Although H5N1 human infections predominated, other human infections with H7 and H9 avian influenza viruses have also been identified. The notoriously unstable genetic nature of influenza viruses makes it impossible to predict which, if any, of these avian influenza viruses will be the cause of the next pandemic and, if so, when that pandemic might occur.

By the end of 2004, it was clear that H5N1 was an especially tenacious virus in avian populations. Tens of millions of birds in many countries were destroyed as part of the control strategy. In large parts of Asia, the virus was firmly entrenched. It was estimated that up to a decade would be required to eliminate it. The threat of a pandemic would also persist, possibly for just as long (Figure 4.2).

As far as humans were concerned, 72% of those infected with H5N1 had died by the end of 2004, with infections still confined to Viet Nam and Thailand. The age profile of cases was disturbing, given that those most frequently infected were previously healthy children and young adults who had been in contact with sick or dead chickens. Most severe cases died following the development of primary viral

Figure 4.2 Cumulative number of confirmed human cases of avian influenza A/(H5N1) reported to WHO since 2003

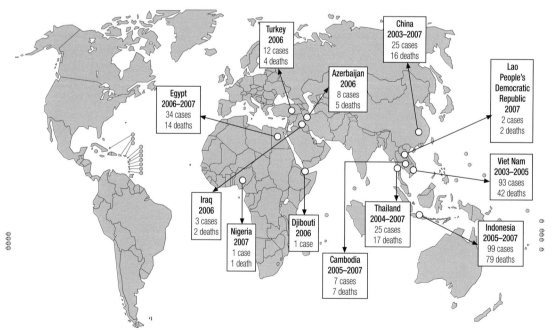

Total number of cases includes number of deaths.
WHO reports only laboratory-confirmed cases.
All dates refer to onset of illness.
Data as of 6 June 2007.

pneumonia, not from super-infections of bacteria which are among the complications of seasonal influenza.

In 2005, so-called "relay transmission" of H5N1 began to occur, with the highly pathogenic virus moving from poultry to wild birds and back again, giving it an ability to move over long distances. In July 2005, the virus moved beyond its initial home in South-East Asia and began to spread, reaching the African continent, Central Asia, Europe and the Eastern Mediterranean Region. With wild birds now involved in the transmission cycle, the prospects for rapid containment of the virus looked even bleaker.

WHO tracked and verified rumours of human cases that reached more than 30 per day. Field investigation kits were dispatched to WHO country offices, and training on field investigations and response was intensified. The GOARN mechanism was mobilized to support the deployment of WHO response teams to 10 countries, while over 30 assessment teams investigated the situation in other countries.

In September 2006, WHO convened a meeting of leading scientists conducting research on the H5N1 virus to consider whether it or another avian influenza virus would retain its exceptional lethality if it acquired the ability to spread efficiently from human to human. It was concluded that, if a pandemic virus emerged following a "reassortment event" – when genetic material is exchanged between human and avian viruses – it would almost certainly lose some of its pathogenicity. However, if the pandemic virus remained entirely avian, yet acquired the ability to transmit from human to human by mutation, it could very well maintain its present lethality. The death rate during the 1918–1919 influenza pandemic was around 2.5%. At 1 May 2007, the overall death rate among reported human H5N1 infections was above 58%.

By 11 April 2007, 12 countries in Asia, the Middle East and Africa had reported the total of human cases and deaths from H5N1 infection given at the beginning of this section. Of these, 28 cases – including 14 deaths – were reported in the first months of 2007, most of them in Egypt (20 cases, including four deaths) and Indonesia (six cases, including five deaths). The outbreaks in poultry continued, as did sporadic cases in humans, but a pandemic virus failed to emerge. Belief began to grow that the threat of a pandemic had been exaggerated. WHO was no longer consistently receiving the information it needed to assess the level of risk and advise the world accordingly. Nevertheless, the threat of a pandemic persists.

Many lessons have been learned from the global response to the pandemic alert. First, the response of countries affected by the virus demonstrated a sense of responsibility and accountability to the international community. This was undoubtedly born of an understanding that, should a country's mismanagement of an outbreak result in the emergence of a pandemic virus, every country in the world would suffer.

Second, the inability of affected countries to sustain an emergency response system over months, if not years, has emerged as an important obstacle to adequate monitoring and assessment of risk. Two assumptions were made at the start of the outbreaks in humans and poultry for the purpose of public health planning: that a pandemic was likely to start quickly and that drastic control measures in poultry would reduce that risk. While not unfounded, both assumptions proved false. Almost no affected country was in a position to sustain the response, initially so intensive, to a protracted emergency. Many other countries introduced appropriate emergency measures at the outset, but could not sustain them. In many cases, countries with limited resources were simply exhausted by the continuing demands of tackling such a tenacious virus in birds and such a treacherous one for humans. Nonetheless, the need for monitoring and assessment remains. International cooperation in identifying all human cases

world health report 2007
global public health security
in the 21st century

50

and sharing the viruses that cause them is important in building a complete picture of the epidemiological situation and maintaining the sensitivity of the warning system. Scientists agree that the threat of a pandemic from H5N1 continues and that the question of a pandemic of influenza from this virus or another avian influenza virus is still a matter of when, not if.

In May 2006, the World Health Assembly adopted a resolution calling for immediate voluntary compliance with provisions in IHR (2005) relevant to avian influenza and the related threat of a pandemic (2). Though the Regulations would not come into legal force until June 2007, this move to accelerate partial implementation was both a measure of the level of concern about the pandemic threat and, equally importantly, an indication of the level of confidence in the difference that the revised Regulations would make.

Many activities in risk reduction and preparedness have been started since the early implementation of IHR (2005). It is clear that the most important risk reduction measure is the control of the panzootic – the equivalent of a pandemic in animals – of H5N1 in chickens because, as long as the virus is present in chicken populations, the threat of a pandemic exists. By controlling the pandemic in poultry, the number of sporadic human infections can also be reduced.

The world remains poorly prepared, however, should control measures in poultry not be effective in risk reduction. In that case, and if the H5N1 or another avian influenza virus – currently, there are 16 known H subtypes and five N subtypes – should

Box 4.1 WHO meeting concludes that global stockpiles of H5N1 vaccine are feasible

In April 2007, a WHO meeting on Options for Increasing the Access of Developing Countries to H5N1 and other Potential Pandemic Vaccines brought together country representatives and vaccine manufacturers. All agreed that creating a stockpile of H5N1 vaccine, and separately developing a mechanism to ensure broader access to pandemic influenza vaccine for developing countries in the event of a pandemic, may be feasible.

"We have taken another crucial step forward in ensuring that all countries have access to the benefits of international influenza virus sharing and pandemic vaccine production," said Dr Margaret Chan, Director-General of WHO. "All countries will now be better placed to protect the public health security of their people and the world at large. Such cooperation is welcome and is consistent with the International Health Regulations, which soon come into force."

Representatives of countries that have experienced human H5N1 infections, donor countries, and vaccine manufacturers from industrialized and developing countries agreed that both scientific evidence and international political commitment supported further efforts to examine whether and how to establish a stockpile of H5N1 vaccine and a mechanism for broader access to a vaccine when the next influenza pandemic occurs.

Participants heard that the Strategic Advisory Group of Experts on Immunization (SAGE) had concluded that recent scientific studies on H5 vaccines had shown them to be safe and immunogenic, and that it was realistic to expect that vaccines offering cross protection (against immunologically related but different viruses not contained in the vaccine) could be developed.

The meeting also heard of the willingness of vaccine manufacturers in developed and developing countries to work with WHO to pursue the possibility of an H5N1 vaccine stockpile and a mechanism for broader access to pandemic vaccines. The International Federation of Pharmaceutical Manufacturers and Associations (IFPMA), representing research-based pharmaceutical companies, forecast increased manufacturing capacity for seasonal influenza vaccines in the next three to five years, to meet potential growing demand.

As a result of the meeting, WHO will set up expert groups to focus on the details of how to create, maintain, fund and use an H5N1 vaccine stockpile, and will continue to consult with appropriate partners and Member States on the development of mechanisms for broader access to pandemic vaccine.

Participants agreed that the work on virus sharing, H5N1 vaccine stockpiles, access to pandemic vaccines and other means of strengthening pandemic preparedness must all be based on IHR (2005).

mutate into a pandemic form, and an early focus of human-to-human transmission be detected before widespread infection occurs, an attempt would be made to contain a pandemic using an antiviral drug. WHO, the Association of South-East Asian Nations (ASEAN) and the United States, among others, have created international stockpiles of oseltamivir, the antiviral drug that potentially could stop transmission in an early focus of human-to-human transmission. WHO has conducted regional workshops to develop preparedness for early containment should it be feasible to intervene, understanding that these measures might not prove effective in stopping or even in slowing the initial spread of a pandemic.

The strategic action proposed by WHO is linked to the six phases of pandemic alert. Currently, the world is at phase three: denoting very limited or no human-to-human transmission. Changes from one phase to another are triggered by several factors, which include the epidemiological behaviour of the disease and the characteristics of circulating viruses. A change from phase three to phase four would result in the rapid containment measures described above.

A shortfall in influenza vaccine production capacity is another reason for the world's inadequate preparedness in case of a pandemic. The current maximum annual production capacity of trivalent seasonal influenza vaccines is 500 million doses, which currently satisfies demand. A greater production capacity would be needed should a pandemic vaccine be required. Consequently, WHO has developed the Global Action Plan for Pandemic Influenza Vaccines to increase the world's production capacity, which would then be available if a pandemic vaccine were required against H5N1 or other avian influenza viruses.

Presently, vaccine manufacturers are producing H5N1 vaccines based on strains of H5N1 that have been selected by WHO. The Global Influenza Surveillance Network described earlier permits selection of those H5N1 viruses because of the free-sharing of these viruses and other avian influenza viruses that infect humans, in addition to the sharing of seasonal influenza viruses.

The free-sharing of H5N1 influenza viruses permits genetic characterization in order to determine the strain of each H5N1 virus and its prevalence in humans; development of non-commercial diagnostic tests for use in public health laboratories around the world in order to assure diagnosis of H5N1 infection; and provision of the most important viruses to vaccine manufacturers and regulatory agencies for the development of H5N1 vaccines.

Furthermore, the free-sharing of H5N1 viruses is critical in risk assessment and risk management under IHR (2005) because, without it, effective global preparedness and global public health security are compromised. Once again, the importance of collaboration in an interconnected world is clearly demonstrated.

Evidence is being collected to determine whether H5N1 vaccines currently under development provide widespread immunity against the three different families of H5N1 virus that currently infect humans, all of them mutations from the original H5N1 virus. This and other scientific evidence are being analysed by WHO to determine, first, whether H5N1 vaccines could be used as preventive vaccines in the same way as current seasonal vaccines; second, whether these types of vaccines would have any value in preventing infection or severe illness should a human pandemic virus develop from H5N1; and third, whether these vaccines should be used, along with antiviral drugs, in an attempt to contain an early focus of human-to-human transmission (see Box 4.1).

WHO's strategic action plan for pandemic influenza

In order to assist countries to prepare for an impending pandemic influenza, WHO developed a strategic action plan for pandemic influenza and works with countries to assess preparedness and response needs. It clearly sets out five key action areas.

- Reducing human exposure to the H5N1 virus.
- Strengthening the early warning system.
- Intensifying rapid containment operations.
- Building capacity to cope with a pandemic.
- Coordinating global scientific research and development.

By 1 May 2007, nearly all countries had established an avian and human pandemic preparedness plan based on the major areas under the WHO plan. This is an impressive and encouraging response. Moreover, WHO has undertaken over 50 missions to support countries experiencing outbreaks of human cases of avian influenza and to assist in laboratory testing and specimen collection, epidemiological investigations, surveillance and risk assessment, social mobilization and outbreak communications, clinical care and infection control, and logistics.

Multi-agency coordination and action within the United Nations system are key elements in supporting countries. The fact that over 70% of new and emerging diseases originate in animals requires a deeper level of cooperation between animal and human health sectors at national and international levels. With the aim of strengthening the coherence of preparedness against avian influenza and a potential human influenza pandemic, the United Nations System Influenza Coordination (UNSIC) was established in 2005. UNSIC's primary responsibility is to respond to government requests for coordinated and sustained international support to implement avian and human influenza programmes, with emphasis placed on the synergy of the contributions made by individual United Nations agencies (*3*).

EXTENSIVELY DRUG-RESISTANT TUBERCULOSIS

Emergence of XDR-TB is a good example of the need for strong health systems to improve public health security, because it is essentially a man-made problem. It is created primarily by inadequate health systems and the resulting failures in programme management, especially poor supervision of health staff and of patients' treatment regimens, disruptions in drug supplies, and poor clinical management, all of which can prevent patients completing courses of treatment.

From January 2005 to March 2006, 221 cases of multidrug-resistant tuberculosis (MDR-TB) were identified at the district hospital in Tugela Ferry, KwaZulu-Natal Province, South Africa. As many as 44 out of 53 patients who were further diagnosed with XDR-TB were also found to be HIV positive. Half of these patients had never previously received treatment for tuberculosis. The mortality rate was extremely high – 52 of the patients died within a median of 16 days of initial sputum collection, of whom two were health workers and 15 were receiving antiretroviral therapy for HIV treatment (*4*).

Widespread infection with HIV provides fertile ground for the transmission of all forms of tuberculosis. The concentration of HIV-infected people in hospitals and, in particular, in antiretroviral treatment programmes, without sufficient measures to control transmission of airborne infections, is enhancing the risk of catching both drug-susceptible and drug-resistant forms of tuberculosis. Health-care workers' reluctance to disclose their positive HIV status to their supervisors may also be putting their own lives at increased risk. In the presence of HIV, untreated tuberculosis will cause death in weeks. The resistant form, even if treated with first-line drugs can, in effect, be considered to be untreated. This was the cause of the extremely high mortality in the cases in KwaZulu-Natal Province.

Beyond the immediate consequences to the affected individuals, the global public health concern is that XDR-TB is as transmissible as its treatable counterparts. Although more study is needed, early research supports these suspicions. In any case, it is of paramount importance that all tuberculosis infections are identified and treated promptly, and that patients complete medication regimens. As of 1 May 2007, XDR–TB has been confirmed in 37 countries, including all G8 member countries.

The management of lesser forms of drug resistance is crucial. If so-called second-line drugs used for treating resistant tuberculosis are not properly supervised, the development of XDR-TB from MDR-TB is only a matter of time. Teams specifically trained in the management of drug resistance and working in dedicated hospitals or isolation units within larger hospitals are essential, as are sufficient beds and a regular supply of high quality second-line drugs.

The neglect of tuberculosis as a major contributor to morbidity and mortality is probably one cause of this category of threats to public health security. Other causes include the global and national policy environments, the quality (or lack of quality) of national tuberculosis control programmes (especially in case management and the implementation of infection control measures) and the prevalence of HIV infection.

None of these conditions is confined to South Africa. Nevertheless, XDR-TB in South Africa is a wake-up call to all countries, and especially those in Africa, to ensure that basic tuberculosis control reaches international standards and to initiate and strengthen management of drug-resistant forms of the disease. Preparedness to respond to XDR-TB includes the provision of laboratories capable of carrying out drug susceptibility testing, which requires the training of clinical and laboratory staff to ensure early diagnosis and a secure supply of high quality second-line drugs. Surveys to determine the geographical spread of MDR-TB and XDR-TB are essential and have the added advantage of providing governments and the media with information on where to issue appropriate messages to the public as well as health-care staff to support correct management, rather than inappropriate enforcement of quarantine and isolation.

The XDR-TB episode is symptomatic of a wider problem affecting many countries, namely, that multiple threats to public health security often have to be dealt with simultaneously. In this case, the tuberculosis crisis is compounded not just by the weakness of control programmes. There is the additional risk of coinfection with HIV, among both patients and health workers who may be in close contact in hospitals and clinics, which are in turn beset by shortages of clinical and laboratory staff and equipment. These deficits are themselves a problem common to many countries and reflect the multiple weaknesses of health systems, particularly in developing countries. In such circumstances, local issues of health security rapidly become national, regional and international. At the international level, the need to attack multi-drug resistance with vigour and urgency was recognized in the Global Plan to Stop TB 2006-2015, but these most recent events have made those working in the field of tuberculosis move to accelerate their global response to drug resistance, particularly in Africa.

As the XDR-TB epidemic continues, an additional mechanism – IHR (2005) – will play an increasingly important role through assessment of its importance as a public health emergency of international concern and a potential collective response.

MANAGING THE RISKS AND CONSEQUENCES OF THE INTERNATIONAL SPREAD OF POLIO

Polio is one of the four internationally notifiable diseases specifically listed in IHR (2005). The 2003-2006 international spread of poliovirus was a wake-up call to a world expecting to bid farewell to polio. While inadequate control (as described in Chapter 2) played a catalytic role in that outbreak, the application of IHR (2005) to a similar situation in the future might greatly facilitate a timely response and substantially reduce the public health consequences.

For the purpose of polio eradication, an extensive infrastructure has been established to enable weekly surveillance and performance monitoring in every country of the world, immediate notification of confirmed polio cases, and ongoing standardized clinical and virologic investigation of potential cases. This infrastructure consists of human resources, standards, operating procedures and physical assets. Formal surveillance reports are now filed weekly from 180 countries, 66% of which have integrated routine reporting of other vaccine-preventable and epidemic-prone diseases. Of the 145 institutions housing laboratories that are part of the polio network, over 85%

Figure 4.3 Poliovirus importations, 2003–2006*

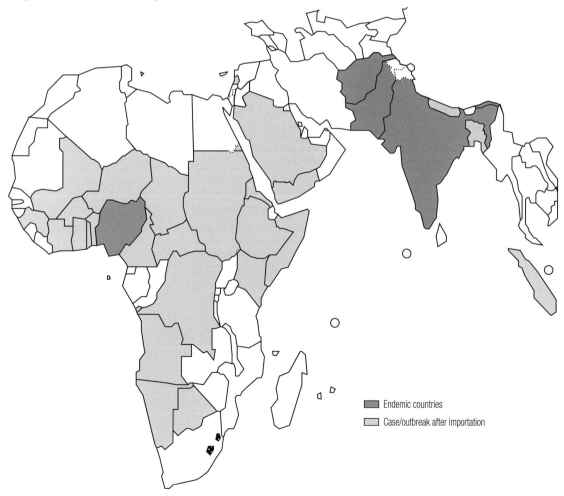

Endemic countries
Case/outbreak after importation

* All cases in Niger from 2005 onward are importation related.

perform analyses for other diseases, such as influenza, measles, meningitis, rubella, and yellow fever.

Given progress towards the goal of global polio eradication and the risk of polio reintroduction or re-emergence in a post-eradication world, long-term surveillance for polioviruses takes on a new importance. The designation of polio in IHR (2005) will further help to prevent, control and interrupt the international spread of the disease in the event of an outbreak during and after eradication. As IHR (2005) comes into force, countries will be assessing their capacity to identify, verify and control circulating wild polioviruses.

The poliovirus has repeatedly shown its ability to travel great distances and enter polio-free areas by land, sea or air travel (see Figure 4.3). In order to minimize the risk and consequences of potential future importations, countries are protecting themselves by maintaining high population immunity and surveillance. The alert and reporting mechanisms mandated by IHR (2005) are an essential complement to these routine immunization activities, particularly for a disease that can circulate without causing symptoms for weeks and has lifelong consequences. This capacity to remain alert and to respond is fundamental to our ability to eradicate polio. It will become doubly so once the virus is eradicated in nature and the world has to guard against the accidental or deliberate release of the virus from facilities where it is being used for research and diagnostics or for the production and quality-control of vaccines.

Looking ahead, it is clear that acute threats to global health security, such as those witnessed in the last years of the 20th century and the first years of this century, will continue to occur, recur or emerge as the world becomes more complex and interconnected and as the microbial world evolves and adapts its virulence, modes of transmission and resistance to drugs in line with its changing environment.

A safer world, therefore, needs a global system based on strong national public health infrastructure and capacity, preparedness and risk reduction for specific health threats, and an effective international system for coordinated alert and response.

Much progress has been made but this cannot be reproduced or sustained without major investments in national, regional and global public health infrastructure.

REFERENCES

1. *FluNet: global influenza programme.* Geneva, World Health Organization, 2003 (http://gamapserver.who.int/GlobalAtlas/home.asp, accessed 1 May 2007).
2. *World Health Assembly agrees to immediate voluntary implementation of influenza-related provisions of International Health Regulations (2005).* Geneva, World Health Organization, 2006 (http://www.who.int/mediacentre/news/releases/2006/wha02/en/index.html, accessed 30 April 2007).
3. *Enhancing capacity building in global public health. Note by the Secretary-General.* New York, NY, United Nations, September 2006 (61st Session of the General Assembly).
4. Gandi NR, Moll A, Sturm AW, Pawinski R, Govender T, Lalloo U et al. Extensively drug-resistant tuberculosis as a cause of death in patients co-infected with tuberculosis and HIV in a rural area of South Africa. *Lancet*, 2006, 368:1575–1580.

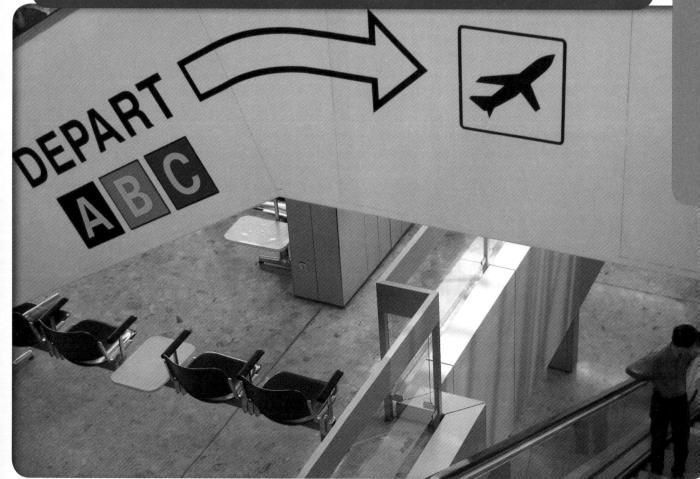

TOWARDS A SAFER FUTURE

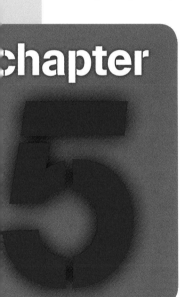

Chapter 5 emphasizes the importance of strengthening health systems in building global public health security. It argues that many of the public health emergencies described in this report could have been prevented or better controlled if the health systems concerned had been stronger and better prepared. Some countries find it more difficult than others to confront threats to public health security effectively because they lack the necessary resources, because their health infrastructure has collapsed as a consequence of under-investment and shortages of trained health workers, or because the infrastructure has been damaged or destroyed by armed conflict or a previous natural disaster. With rare exceptions, threats to public health are generally known and manageable.

The world has, after all, accumulated the knowledge and experience of centuries of confronting such dangers. The evolution of measures such as quarantine, sanitation and immunization, outlined in Chapter 1, the rapid scientific and technological advances of the late 20th century, and flourishing international partnerships in health that use the latest communications have together led to a much better understanding of important public health events in today's globalized world.

Chapter 2 gave examples of the tragic and costly consequences of inadequate health system investment, surveillance and control, as in the case of AIDS, dengue and other infectious diseases; and Chapter 4 provided a further example in the case of extensively drug-resistant tuberculosis. Strengthening health systems is a continuous priority for WHO. As discussed at length in *The World Health Report 2006 – Working together for health*, many national health systems today are weak, unresponsive, inequitable and even unsafe. The 2006 report identified 57 countries where shortages are so dire that they are very unlikely in the near future to be able to provide high coverage of essential interventions. These shortages are equivalent to a global deficit of 2.4 million doctors, nurses and midwives.

These 57 countries, most of them in sub-Saharan Africa and South-East Asia, are struggling to provide even basic health security to their populations. How, then, can they be expected to become a part of an unbroken line of defence, employing the most up-to-date technologies, upon which global public health security depends?

Such a defence is reliant on strong national public health systems that are well-equipped – both with appropriate technology and talented and dedicated personnel – to detect, investigate, communicate and contain events that threaten public health security whenever and wherever they occur.

Clearly, the strengthening of weaker health systems is essential not only to assure the best possible public health of national populations, but also to assure global public health security. These national and international priorities are welded together by IHR (2005), which call for national core capacity strengthening and collective global action for public health emergencies of international concern – those events that endanger global public health.

HELPING COUNTRIES HELPS THE WORLD

The examples of avian influenza, extensively drug-resistant tuberculosis and poliomyelitis, given in Chapter 4, represent current threats to national and international public health security – each event should prompt the relevant country to apply the decision instrument of IHR (2005) (see Figure 5.1).

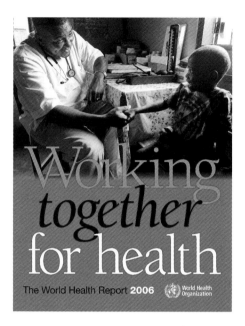

If an event falls within the requirements of the decision instrument, and is confirmed to be a public health emergency of international concern, the country is obliged to report it to WHO. In turn, WHO and its partners will respond as necessary with support to contain the threat at its source. This is, of course, how the Regulations best serve the interests of global public health security in an ideal world. In reality, not all countries have the resources to fully meet the core capacity requirements of the Regulations immediately, or even by the 2012 deadline. They are, therefore, poorly equipped to detect, identify and respond to events, compromising global public health security.

This limitation poses significant challenges to all countries, WHO and its partners in global public health security. The following section explores these challenges and presents strategies to overcome them. Seven strategic actions are set out in Table 5.1 to assist countries with the challenges inherent in meeting the new obligations.

Global partnerships

The success of IHR (2005) depends to a large extent upon strong international partnerships. In many areas, such as in the area of infectious disease and chemical dangers, these partnerships already exist. In others they need to be built. Partnerships between, for example, ministries of health and WHO, are well established and will more easily fall in step with the requirements of IHR (2005).

Less traditional partnerships, such as those between health, travel and defence, will require concerted efforts at the national level to ensure the interests of all parties are transparent and well represented. The IHR (2005) are intended to minimize impact on travel and trade, yet there may be times when difficult decisions will have to be made that will affect these sectors. Strong partnerships, a full understanding of IHR (2005), and the urgent need to halt the international spread of disease in the best interests of economies as well as public health will facilitate such decisions.

Part of the challenge when creating and maintaining effective partnerships is in building trust from various perspectives: trusting individual countries to change mindsets and move from covering up disease outbreaks to adopting transparency from the initial case or event, and trusting WHO to act on information in the world's best interests, while minimizing the impact on the economy of reporting countries.

WHO must, of course, earn this trust through country support during the initial assessment and ongoing implementation phases of IHR (2005), and through open dialogue with governments, private sector institutions, funding organizations, partner United Nations agencies and civil society.

Trust between countries is also critical in establishing the highest level of global health security possible. All 193 WHO Member States are parties to IHR (2005), but not all currently have the capacity requirements to implement them fully. Technical and financial assistance, beyond that provided by WHO, will be necessary. Bilateral agreements will be built on the understanding that failure in one country is a threat to all, and global benefits can only come from mutual cooperation.

Figure 5.1 Events that may constitute a public health emergency of international concern: the decision instrument*

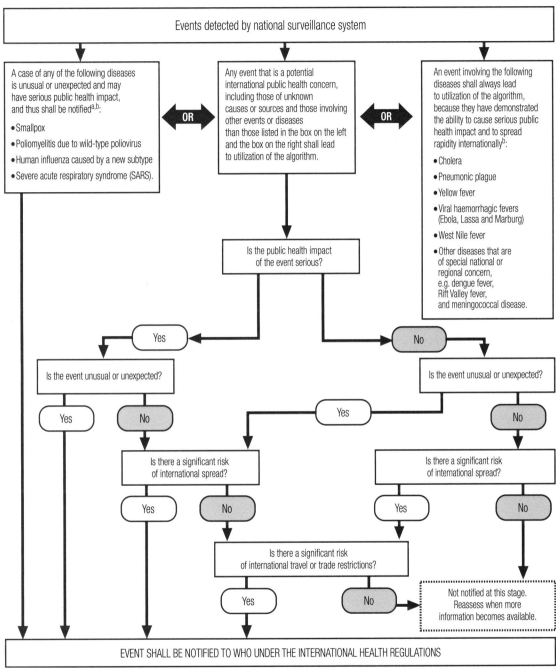

* Extracted from Annex II of IHR (2005).

[a] As per WHO case definitions. [b] The disease list shall be used only for the purposes of these Regulations.

Table 5.1 Seven strategic actions to guide IHR (2005) implementation[a]

	Strategic action	Goal
GLOBAL PARTNERSHIP		
1	**Foster global partnerships**	WHO, all countries and all relevant sectors (e.g. health, agriculture, travel, trade, education, defence) are aware of the new rules and collaborate to provide the best available technical support and, where needed, mobilize the necessary resources for effective implementation of IHR (2005).
STRENGTHEN NATIONAL CAPACITY		
2	**Strengthen national disease surveillance, prevention, control and response systems**	Each country assesses its national resources in disease surveillance and response and develops national action plans to implement and meet IHR (2005) requirements, thus permitting rapid detection and response to the risk of international disease spread.
3	**Strengthen public health security in travel and transport**	The risk of international spread of disease is minimized through effective permanent public health measures and response capacity at designated airports, ports and ground crossings in all countries.
PREVENT AND RESPOND TO INTERNATIONAL PUBLIC HEALTH EMERGENCIES		
4	**Strengthen WHO global alert and response systems**	Timely and effective coordinated response to international public health risks and public health emergencies of international concern.
5	**Strengthen the management of specific risks**	Systematic international and national management of the risks known to threaten international health security, such as influenza, meningitis, yellow fever, SARS, poliomyelitis, food contamination, chemical and radioactive substances.
LEGAL ISSUES AND MONITORING		
6	**Sustain rights, obligations and procedures**	New legal mechanisms as set out in the Regulations are fully developed and upheld; all professionals involved in implementing IHR (2005) have a clear understanding of, and sustain, the new rights, obligations and procedures laid out in the Regulations.
7	**Conduct studies and monitor progress**	Indicators are identified and collected regularly to monitor and evaluate IHR (2005) implementation at national and international levels. WHO Secretariat reports on progress to the World Health Assembly. Specific studies are proposed to facilitate and improve implementation of the Regulations.

[a] Strategic actions 2–5 are key because they call for significantly strengthened national and global efforts.

Strengthening national capacity

National, intermediary and local public health systems are charged with providing the core capacities needed to detect, assess, report and deploy rapid control measures to public health events of international concern. In line with the Regulations, Member States must complete an initial assessment of their capacity to meet these require-ments by the June 2009 deadline, and, if found insufficient, develop a national plan to build the necessary capacity within the following three years. Several countries began capacity building and implementation of the Regulations before they entered into force (see Box 5.1). For many more countries, financial and human resources constraints will hamper their ability to meet the deadline. WHO has a critical role to play in assisting countries to build capacity and estimates that it will have to support 115 countries to develop national plans of action or strategy papers to meet the Regulations' core capacity requirements (*1*).

Box 5.1 IHR (2005) – early implementation efforts

Global Partnerships

The Andean Health Organization (Organismo Andino de Salud), an institution of the Andean Integration System, coordinates and supports the efforts made by its mem-ber countries, both individually and jointly, to improve the health of their people.

During the March 2007 meeting of the Ministries of Health, it was decided to merge all the existing surveillance networks in South America and to create a regional network for surveillance and response in order to harmonize the instruments and processes in the member states (*2*).

Several countries have also set up Emergency Opera-tion Centers (EOC) that will enable them to physically as well as virtually centralize the epidemic intelligence and the coordination of the response to a real or a potential emergency. The EOC will have the responsibility to obtain, organize, analyse, prioritize, monitor and disseminate information about health emergencies.

A number of countries – Argentina, Brazil, Canada, Mexico, Peru and the United States – have already set up EOCs and will support, in collaboration with the WHO Regional Office for the Americas, other countries in the region to establish additional centres. In conjunction with the National IHR Focal Points, EOCs will constitute a pow-erful infrastructure for alert and response to public health emergencies.

National capacity building

In anticipation of the coming into force of IHR (2005), the Kingdom of Morocco has begun activities to strengthen the competencies of health professionals involved in the application of the Regulations and is progressively put-ting in place the necessary tools and means to strengthen the core capacity requirements for surveillance and response.

Ongoing workshops and technical training for air-port and port health officers were initiated in 2007. Areas covered include a review of the information system of airport and port health authorities; the adap-tation of existing health documents to the new models set out in IHR (2005); and comprehensive strengthening of public health capacities at designated international points of entry.

In a commitment to cross-sector collaboration and representation, Morocco has also established an inter-ministerial committee for the implementation of the Regulations. The first meeting of this group symboli-cally coincided with the launch of IHR (2005) on 15 June 2007.

Legal issues

Canada's direct experience with SARS prompted the government to update its Quarantine Act in 2004. At the time, the Act contained elements that could be traced back to 1872, when Canada was a new nation and the primary mode of travel was by sea. It was, therefore, in dire need of modernization. A new Quarantine Act was passed by the Parliament of Canada in May 2005 and came into force on 12 December 2006, seven months prior to the implementation of IHR (2005).

The revision of the new Quarantine Act ran in par-allel with the development of the revised Regulations, with their respective adoptions in May and June 2005. Although the simultaneous development provided the opportunity for insights, there are some IHR (2005) obligations, primarily concerning points of entry, which were not reflected in the new Quarantine Act. The government is currently reviewing those gaps and will be proposing amendments to meet the core capacity requirements of the Regulations.

National plans will vary from country to country, but will contain components such as building or strengthening national public health institutes; ensuring that national surveillance and response systems use internationally recognized quality standards; strengthening human resources capacity through training programmes in intervention epidemiology, outbreak investigation, laboratory diagnostics, case management, infection control, social mobilization and risk communication; and using WHO indicators to carry out regular assessments of core capacities to monitor progress and assess future needs. In this regard, WHO expects the number of countries participating in training programmes related to IHR (2005) core capacities to increase from 100 in 2008 to 150 in 2009 (1).

The control of diseases at border crossings – whether land, sea or air – is an essential element of the Regulations. Many of the requirements for protecting public health apply to these locations and are new or different from the previous Regulations. They will require close collaboration between WHO and other organizations of the United Nations system (e.g. the International Civil Aviation Organization (ICAO), the International Maritime Organization (IMO) and the World Tourism Organization (UNWTO)) and professional associations (e.g. the International Air Transport Association (IATA) and the Airports Council International (ACI)). Contingency plans for public health emergencies and the capacity to implement them must be available at all designated points of entry in all countries.

Some countries will find it more difficult than others to confront threats to public health security effectively. This may be because they lack the necessary resources and technical capacity, because their health infrastructure has collapsed as a consequence of under-investment and shortages of trained health workers, or because the infrastructure has been damaged or destroyed by armed conflict or a previous natural disaster.

In addition to a strengthened alert and response capacity component, the Regulations also legally bind WHO to support countries in building their capacity to meet their obligations under IHR (2005). Work includes facilitating national and international resource mobilization and advocacy. These activities are especially crucial for the countries that have the weakest health systems. Health crises of epidemics, natural disasters and conflict are often unexpected and can quickly overwhelm national health systems, especially those already in a precarious state.

During public health emergencies, local communities are the first to respond, followed by district and national governments. Many societies do not have the resources to be adequately prepared at all times, and countries do not always have the resources to manage a major emergency or outbreak without external assistance. Qualified, experienced, and well-prepared international health personnel are often needed to help. Cooperation between countries is necessary to ensure the safety net provided for in IHR (2005), as described in Chapter 1. The quality of response, ultimately, depends upon workforce preparedness based on local capacity backed by timely international support.

Well-prepared health systems can effectively contribute to preventing health events from becoming security emergencies. Many newly emerging security scenarios, such as deliberate releases of chemical, biological or radionuclear substances and potential terrorist attacks, are intended to jeopardize the health and security of communities, with health services being the first entry point for possible victims. In the first instance, such health emergencies might not immediately be recognized as a security event, particularly if health systems are inadequately prepared for – or unaware of – such potential scenarios. It is crucial to promote further collaboration and a continuous dialogue between health professionals, security officials and policy-makers to increase mutual understanding of respective systems and operational procedures.

Preventing and responding to international public health emergencies

No single country – however capable, wealthy or technologically advanced – can alone prevent, detect and respond to all public health threats. Emerging threats may be unseen from a national perspective, may require a global analysis for proper risk assessment, and may necessitate effective coordination at the international level.

This is the basis for the revised Regulations. As not all countries are able to take up the challenge immediately, WHO is drawing upon its long experience as the leader in global public health, its convening power, and its partnerships with governments, United Nations agencies, civil society, academia, the private sector and the media to maintain its surveillance and global alert and response systems.

As described in Chapter 1, WHO surveillance networks, (e.g. GOARN, ChemiNet, the polio surveillance network) are effective international partnerships that provide both a service and a safety net. GOARN, for example, is able to deploy response teams to any part of the world within 24 hours to provide direct support to national authorities. WHO's various surveillance and laboratory networks are able to capture the global picture of public health risks and assist in efficient case analysis (see Figure 5.2). Together, these systems fill acute gaps caused by the lack of national capacity and protect the world when there may be a desire to delay reporting for political or other reasons.

The effective maintenance of these systems, however, must be adequately resourced with staff, technology and financial support. The building of national capacity will not diminish the need for WHO's global networks. Rather, increased partnerships, knowledge transfer, advancing technologies, event management and strategic communications will grow as IHR (2005) reaches full implementation.

Figure 5.2 Verified events of potential international public health concern, by WHO region, September 2003–September 2006

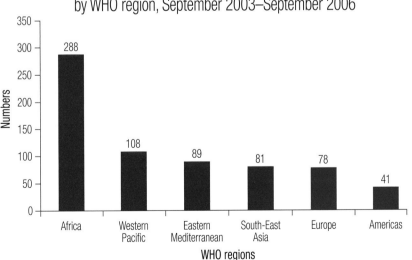

Total number of cases = 685

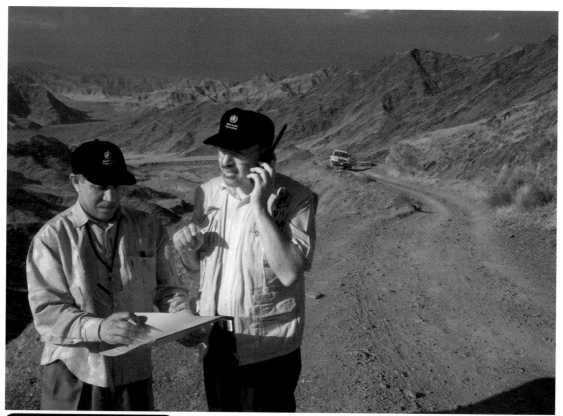

WHO emergency response teams deploy to even the most remote regions within 24 hours

Simultaneous with the need to prepare for urgent response is the need to prevent and contain the diseases and other incidents that could cause a public health crisis warranting international response. As mentioned previously, medical personnel working on prevention programmes, such as polio immunization campaigns, are often the first point of entry into the public health system and can detect the earliest suspicious cases of disease, food safety outbreak, chemical exposure or other threatening situation. For the obvious benefit of prevention, particularly of those diseases that either automatically require notification under IHR (2005) – such as polio due to wild-type poliovirus, or SARS – or those that always require the use of the decision instrument (e.g. cholera, pneumonic plague or yellow fever) it is important to maintain and strengthen WHO's international disease control programmes.

Legal issues and monitoring

It is not only public health professionals working in clinics and laboratories who must understand the new requirements under IHR (2005). Policy-makers and national public health officials must appreciate the new legal requirements agreed to by all parties and, if necessary, take action to bring national policies in line with them. Canada, for example, revised its Quarantine Act in parallel with the development of IHR (2005) (see Box 5.1).

While the Regulations are not unknown to countries, the shift in conceptual framework – from control at borders to containment at the source; from a list of diseases to all public health threats; from preset measures to an adapted response – will require a shift in understanding that will take time to assimilate.

In order to ensure that understanding grows in line with the technical aspects of implementation, WHO is developing specialized training programmes for legal and public health professionals and is assisting countries to adapt or develop existing or new public health legislation to comply with the Regulations.

The only way to ensure understanding of and compliance with the revised IHR (2005) is to actively monitor the progress of implementation efforts at the national, regional and global levels. Feedback, particularly during the initial phases, will provide insight into areas for improvement in training, implementation and adherence strategies. It should also serve to build donors' confidence in the capacity of WHO and recipient countries to execute the core capacities of IHR (2005) with rigour and efficiency.

WHO is charged with making regular assessment reports to the World Health Assembly that will include quantitative and qualitative measures of progress and difficulties encountered in implementation at all levels, including national public health systems and legal procedures and processes, as well as proposals for research areas, recommendations to improve implementation and ongoing resource requirements.

REFERENCES

1. *Medium-term strategic plan 2008–2013 and proposed programme budget 2008–2009*. Geneva, World Health Organization, 2007.
2. *Resolución XXVIII/428: Resoluciones de la XXVIII Reunión Ordinaria de Ministros de Salud del Area Andina, Santa Cruz de la Sierra, Bolivia, 29 y 30 Marzo del 2007* [Resolution XXVIII/428: Resolutions of the XXVIII Ordinary Meeting of Ministers of Health of the Andean Region, Santa Cruz de la Sierra, Bolivia, 29–30 March 2007]. Lima, Organismo Andino de Salud, 2007.

66

world health report 2007
global public health security
in the 21st century

CONCLUSIONS & RECOMMENDATIONS

It cannot be over-emphasized that a truly effective international preparedness and response coordination mechanism cannot be managed nationally. Global cooperation, collaboration and investment are necessary to ensure a safer future. This means a multi-sectoral approach to managing the problem of global disease that includes governments, industry, public and private financiers, academia, international organizations and civil society, all of whom have responsibilities for building global public health security.

In achieving the highest level of global public health security possible, it is important that each sector recognizes its global responsibility. The IHR (2005) mandate core capacities for countries and obligations for WHO. They do not oblige other sectors to act in accord. Nonetheless, the building of global public health security rests on a solid foundation of transparent and benevolent partnerships. In the spirit of such partnership, WHO urges all involved to acknowledge their roles and responsibilities for global public health security through the following recommendations:

1 Full implementation of IHR (2005) by all countries. The protection of national and global public health must be transparent in government affairs, be seen as a cross-cutting issue and as a crucial element integrated into economic and social policies and systems.

2 Global cooperation in surveillance and outbreak alert and response between governments, United Nations agencies, private sector industries and organizations, professional associations, academia, media agencies and civil society, building particularly on the eradication of polio to create an effective and comprehensive surveillance and response infrastructure.

3 Open sharing of knowledge, technologies and materials, including viruses and other laboratory samples, necessary to optimize secure global public health. The struggle for global public health security will be lost if vaccines, treatment regimens, and facilities and diagnostics are available only to the wealthy.

Global responsibility for capacity building within the public health infrastructure of all countries. National systems must be strengthened to anticipate and predict hazards effectively both at the international and national levels and to allow for effective preparedness strategies.

 Cross-sector collaboration within governments. The protection of global public health security is dependent on trust and collaboration between sectors such as health, agriculture, trade and tourism. It is for this reason that the capacity to understand and act in the best interests of the intricate relationship between public health security and these sectors must be fostered.

 Increased global and national resources for the training of public health personnel, the advancement of surveillance, the building and enhancing of laboratory capacity, the support of response networks, and the continuation and progression of prevention campaigns.

This report has focused primarily on acute threats to health. In order to ensure a complete spectrum of public health security, however, the discussion would also include endemic threats to health, such as those related to maternal and child health, chronic disease, violence and mental health, among others. These conditions do not meet the notification criteria of IHR (2005), yet they make up the majority of the global burden of death and disability.

Professionals and policy-makers in the fields of public health, foreign policy and national security should maintain open dialogue on endemic diseases and practices that pose personal health threats, including HIV/AIDS, which also have the potential to threaten national and international health security.

Although the subject of *The World Health Report 2007* has taken a global approach to public health, WHO is not neglecting the fact that all individuals – women, men and children – are affected by the common threats to health. It is vital not to lose sight of the personal consequences of global health challenges. This was the inspiration that led to the "health for all" commitment towards primary health care in 1978. That commitment and the principles supporting it remain untarnished and as essential as ever.

On that basis, primary health care and humanitarian action in times of crisis – two means to ensure health security at individual and community levels – will be discussed at length in *The World Health Report 2008*.

index

70

world health report 2007
global public health security
in the 21st century